THE
HUMAN BRAIN
in Photographs and Diagrams

Second Edition

THE
HUMAN BRAIN
in Photographs and Diagrams

Second Edition

JOHN NOLTE, PhD
Professor of Cell Biology and Anatomy
Director, Division of Academic Resources
The University of Arizona College of Medicine
Tucson, Arizona

JAY B. ANGEVINE, JR., PhD
Professor Emeritus of Cell Biology and Anatomy
The University of Arizona College of Medicine
Tucson, Arizona

with 558 illustrations

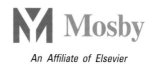
Mosby
An Affiliate of Elsevier

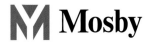

An Affiliate of Elsevier

Editor: William Schmitt
Project Manager: Carol Sullivan Weis
Senior Production Editor: Karen M. Rehwinkel
Designer: Mark A. Oberkrom
Cover Designer: Kathi Gosche

SECOND EDITION
Copyright © 2000 by Mosby, Inc.

Previous editions copyrighted 1995

Mosby, Inc.
An Affiliate of Elsevier
11830 Westline Industrial Drive
St. Louis, Missouri 63146

Printed in China

ISBN-13: 978–0–323–01126–6
ISBN-10: 0–323–01126–8

Last digit is the print number: 9   8   7   6   5   4

To Our Students
whose enthusiasm maintains ours,
whose questions prod us to seek clarity and accuracy,
whose caring and curiosity make teaching fun;

and

To Paul Ivan Yakovlev
whose wisdom and foresight,
dignity, kindness, and generosity,
reverence for patients and joy in people,
enormous energy and personal youthfulness
created a world library of human and animal brains
and a world community of neurological scholars.

Learning about the functional anatomy of the human central nervous system (CNS) is usually a daunting task. Structures that interdigitate and overlap in three dimensions contribute to the difficulty, as does a long list of intimidating names, many with origins in descriptive terminology derived from Latin and Greek. We have attempted in this book to make the task a little easier for students of the biological and health sciences, by presenting systematic series of whole-brain sections in three different sets of planes, by relating these sections to three-dimensional reconstructions, and by trying to restrain ourselves when indicating structures.

We made a number of choices in organizing the materials for the first edition of this atlas, and again in developing the second edition; in each instance we strove for simplicity. Unlabeled photographs are presented throughout the book, juxtaposed to faded-out versions of the same photographs with important structures outlined and labeled. This circumvents the common need to mentally superimpose a labeled drawing on a photograph. We pored over many hundreds of sections and chose what we believe to be comprehensive yet not excessive sets in each plane; sections illustrating major structures or major transitions are shown in color and at a higher magnification. Every labeled structure is discussed briefly in a glossary at the end of the book. New to this edition are several additional views of gross brains (Chapter 1), higher magnification views of parts of the spinal cord and brainstem sections (Chapters 2 and 3), one or two more enlarged color views in most planes of section (Chapters 3, 5, 6, and 7), and brief discussions of the CNS pathways subserving the chemical senses (Chapter 8). We also corrected a few labeling errors that crept into the first edition and added illustrative inserts to some of the pathway diagrams in Chapter 8.

These methods inevitably involve compromises. We labeled only structures that we believe are important for the knowledge base of undergraduate and professional students and omitted others dear to our hearts but perhaps not critical for these students. Hence the fasciola cinerea so prominent in Figure 6-10 is not labeled, and the indusium griseum is mentioned only briefly in a footnote. In addition, explicitly outlining structures required some simplifications, and complex entities are sometimes indicated more simply as single structures. We think the resulting pedagogical utility for students justifies these anatomical liberties.

Current technological methods allowed us to approach the construction of this atlas differently than we could have just a few years ago. All of the photographs of brains and sections used in the book were digitized and then retouched digitally. Mounting medium, staining artifacts, and small cracks, folds, and scratches were removed from the digitized versions of the sections. The profiles of many small blood vessels were removed as well. The color balance was changed as appropriate to make the sections as uniform as possible. These procedures improved the illustrations aesthetically, while leaving their essential content unchanged. In addition, computer-based surface-reconstruction algorithms made possible the beautiful three-dimensional images that appear in Chapter 4 and elsewhere in the book.

Acknowledgments. This book could never have happened without the help of many friends and colleagues. The photographic expertise of Nathan Nitzky and others in the Division of Biomedical Communications is evident throughout the book. Grant Dahmer and Dr. Norman Koelling prepared the prosections shown in Chapter 1. The sections shown in Chapter 2 were cut by Shelley Rowley, and those in Chapter 3 by John Nolte's colleague and friend, Pam Eller. John Sundsten produced the three-dimensional images shown in Chapter 4 and elsewhere in the book and shared in our excitement about this project. Paul Yakovlev, as detailed shortly, was the central figure in the production of the sections shown in Chapters 5 through 7. Drs. Ray Carmody, Art Gmitro, Robert Handy, and Joe Seeger provided the images shown in Chapter 9 and helped with their interpretation. Sasha Zill first described the strumus. Carol and Midge cheered us on. We thank them all.

John Nolte and Jay B. Angevine, Jr.
Tucson, Arizona
February, 2000

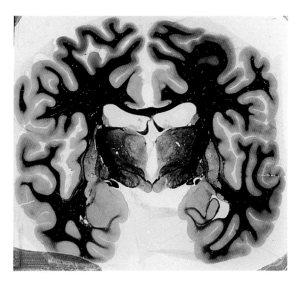

The section shown in Figure 5-7, before retouching.

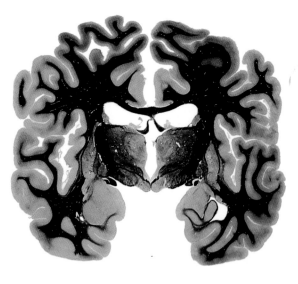

The section shown in Figure 5-7, retouched.

A Note on the Whole-Brain Serial Sections and Their Origin

As crucial as computer technology is to our book, the whole-brain serial sections are its foundation. They were prepared during 1966–1967 in the Warren Anatomical Museum at Harvard Medical School. The work, in which I took part, was performed under the direction of Dr. Paul I. Yakovlev (1894–1983), who was curator of the museum from 1955 to 1961 and then Emeritus Clinical Professor of Neuropathology until 1969. Each brain, embedded whole in celloidin, was sectioned in coronal, horizontal, or sagittal planes on a giant microtome with a standing oblique 36-inch blade and a sliding brain holder. The sections, each 35 micrometers thick, were rolled and stored in test tubes in a console of 100 numbered receptacles. After processing pilot sections for suitability and quality, we stained every 20th section with Weigert's hematoxylin (Loyez method) for myelin and mounted it in window glass. Each preparation is thus about 4 mm thick, yet great depth and detail of cells and fibers are visible in it.

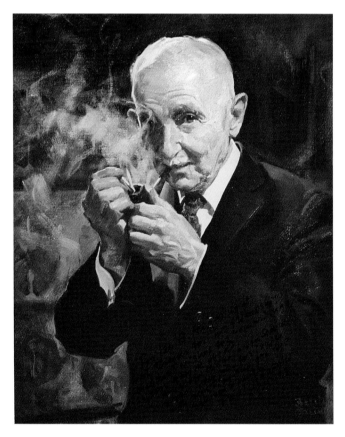

Paul I. Yakovlev, MD
1894–1983
An autographed copy of an oil portrait of Paul Yakovlev by Bettina Steinke. The original portrait was presented to the Warren Anatomical Museum at Harvard Medical School in 1978. (Courtesy of the Warren Museum in the Francis A. Countway Library of Medicine, Boston, Massachusetts.)

Such preparations illustrate the white matter and tracts of the brain by staining the myelin sheaths of axons black; gray matter and nuclei appear as more or less pale areas, depending on the number and caliber of myelinated fibers present. These sections, all from essentially normal brains, were added to an already huge collection representing over 900 cerebra that Dr. Yakovlev had been building since 1930. Now a national resource known and available to neurological scholars world-wide, this priceless compilation known as the Yakovlev Collection is graciously housed by the Armed Forces Institute of Pathology in Washington, DC. Today it comprises about 1600 specimens, normal and pathological, processed in a rigorously consistent manner from the start.

In mid-1967, with Dr. Yakovlev's blessing, I took with me to The University of Arizona some 1000 of the 8741 sections cut from the three normal brains used in Chapters 5 through 7 of this book. I had left Boston to join the faculty of the University's new College of Medicine in Tucson. Paul, my mentor from the time I came to Harvard in 1956, wanted to support me as I began teaching in a far-off land that he believed (perhaps correctly) to be a frontier: the "Wild West." As with everything else he did, it was thoughtful, kind, and generous. How he would have loved to see you studying the sections illustrated on these pages! And were he standing beside you, how much you would learn!

Unlike the fairly simple task of sectioning the brainstem, cutting perfect gapless whole-brain serial sections is difficult. The procedure was never more carefully undertaken or widely employed than by Paul, who used it at or in association with Harvard Medical School for 40 years. A central theme for him was this holistic method ("every part of the brain is there, nothing is left out…"), but no aspect of neuroanatomy or neuropathology failed to intrigue him. Although such sections had been made since the late 19th century (they are found in small numbers at many medical schools and in profusion at a few research institutes), Paul's are unique—in uniformity of preparation at every step from fixation to mounting and in unity of general neurological interest and comparability. Of this legacy (he called it "over 40 tons of glass"), Derek Denny-Brown, Emeritus Professor of Neurology at Harvard, wrote in 1972: "The perspective given by serial whole brain sections provides at once an arresting view of anatomical relationships in patterns of striking beauty. After working in the collection for years one still finds every occasion to view it illuminating and rewarding."

Jay B. Angevine, Jr.

EXTERNAL ANATOMY OF THE BRAIN

This atlas emphasizes views of the interior of the human central nervous system (CNS), sectioned in various planes. This first chapter lays some of the groundwork for understanding the arrangements of these interior structures by presenting the surface features with which they are continuous, and by giving a broad overview of the components of the CNS.

The CNS is composed of the spinal cord and the brain, the major components of which are indicated in Figure 1-1. The human brain is dominated by two very large cerebral hemispheres, separated from each other by a deep longitudinal fissure. Each hemisphere is convoluted externally in a fairly consistent pattern into a series of gyri, separated from each other by a series of sulci (an adaptation that makes more area available for the cortex that covers each cerebral hemisphere). Several prominent sulci are used as major landmarks to divide each hemisphere into five lobes*—frontal, parietal, occipital, temporal, and limbic—each of which contains a characteristic set of gyri (Figures 1-2 to 1-6). The two hemispheres are interconnected by a massive bundle of nerve fibers called the corpus callosum. Finally, certain areas of gray matter are embedded in the interior of each cerebral hemisphere. These include major components of the basal ganglia (or, more properly, basal nuclei) and limbic system (primarily the amygdala and hippocampus). They are apparent in the brain sections shown in Chapters 5 through 7.

The cerebral hemispheres of humans are so massive that they almost conceal the remaining major subdivisions of the brain—the diencephalon, brainstem, and cerebellum. Hemisecting a brain in the midsagittal plane, as in Figure 1-1, *B,* reveals these components.

The diencephalon (literally the "in-between brain") is interposed between each cerebral hemisphere and the brainstem. The diencephalon contains the thalamus, a major way station for information seeking access to the cerebral cortex; the hypothalamus, a major control center for visceral and drive-related functions; and several other structures.

The brainstem, continuous caudally with the spinal cord, serves as a conduit for pathways traveling between the cerebellum or spinal cord and more rostral levels of the CNS. It also contains the neurons that receive or give rise to most of the cranial nerves.

The cerebellum is even more intricately convoluted than the cerebral hemispheres to make room for an extensive covering of its own cortex. It plays a major role in the planning and coordination of movement. A deep transverse fissure (normally occupied over most of its extent by the tentorium cerebelli) separates the cerebellum from the overlying occipital and parietal lobes and then continues deeper into the brain, partially separating the diencephalon from the cerebral hemispheres.

---

*In addition, the insula, an area of cerebral cortex buried deep in the lateral sulcus (see Figure 5-7, *A*) is usually considered as a separate lobe.

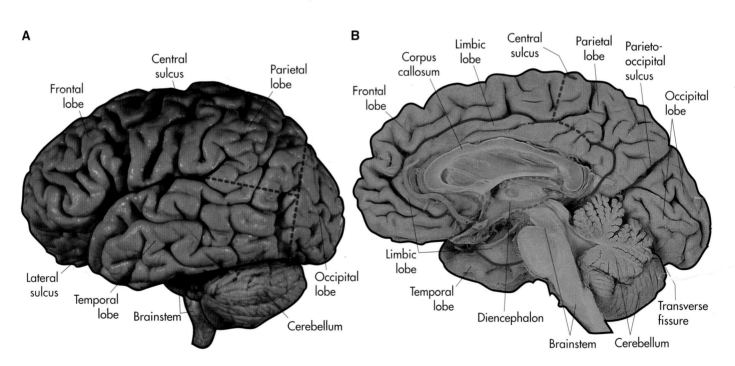

A

Central sulcus

Parietal lobe

Frontal lobe

Lateral sulcus

Temporal lobe   Brainstem

Occipital lobe

Cerebellum

B

Corpus callosum

Limbic lobe

Central sulcus

Parietal lobe

Parieto-occipital sulcus

Frontal lobe

Occipital lobe

Limbic lobe

Temporal lobe

Diencephalon

Brainstem   Cerebellum

Transverse fissure

FIGURE 1-1
Lateral and medial surfaces of the brain, shown slightly less than half actual size. **A,** The left lateral surface of the brain (shown in more detail in Figures 1-3 and 1-6); anterior is to the left. **B,** The medial surface of the right half of the sagittally hemisected brain (shown in more detail in Figure 1-5); anterior is to the left. *(Dissections courtesy of Grant Dahmer, Department of Cell Biology and Anatomy, University of Arizona College of Medicine.)*

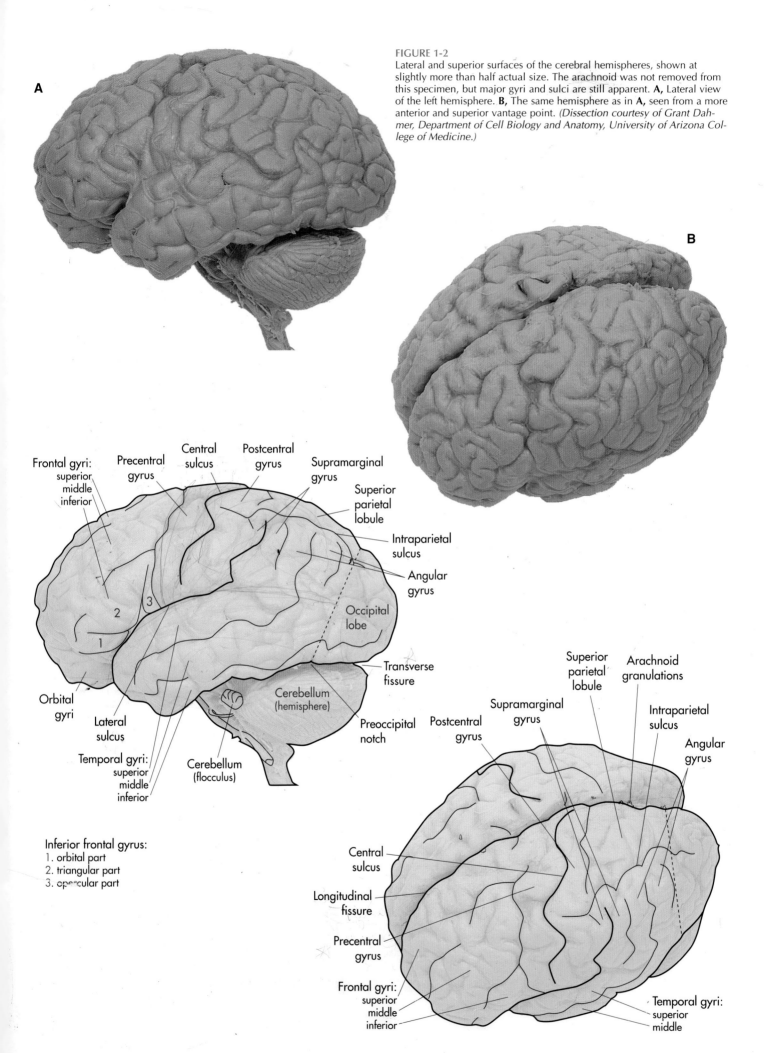

A

B

FIGURE 1-2
Lateral and superior surfaces of the cerebral hemispheres, shown at slightly more than half actual size. The arachnoid was not removed from this specimen, but major gyri and sulci are still apparent. **A,** Lateral view of the left hemisphere. **B,** The same hemisphere as in **A,** seen from a more anterior and superior vantage point. *(Dissection courtesy of Grant Dahmer, Department of Cell Biology and Anatomy, University of Arizona College of Medicine.)*

Frontal gyri:
  superior
  middle
  inferior

Precentral gyrus

Central sulcus

Postcentral gyrus

Supramarginal gyrus

Superior parietal lobule

Intraparietal sulcus

Angular gyrus

Occipital lobe

Transverse fissure

Cerebellum (hemisphere)

Preoccipital notch

Orbital gyri

Lateral sulcus

Temporal gyri:
  superior
  middle
  inferior

Cerebellum (flocculus)

Inferior frontal gyrus:
1. orbital part
2. triangular part
3. opercular part

Superior parietal lobule

Arachnoid granulations

Intraparietal sulcus

Angular gyrus

Supramarginal gyrus

Postcentral gyrus

Central sulcus

Longitudinal fissure

Precentral gyrus

Frontal gyri:
  superior
  middle
  inferior

Temporal gyri:
  superior
  middle

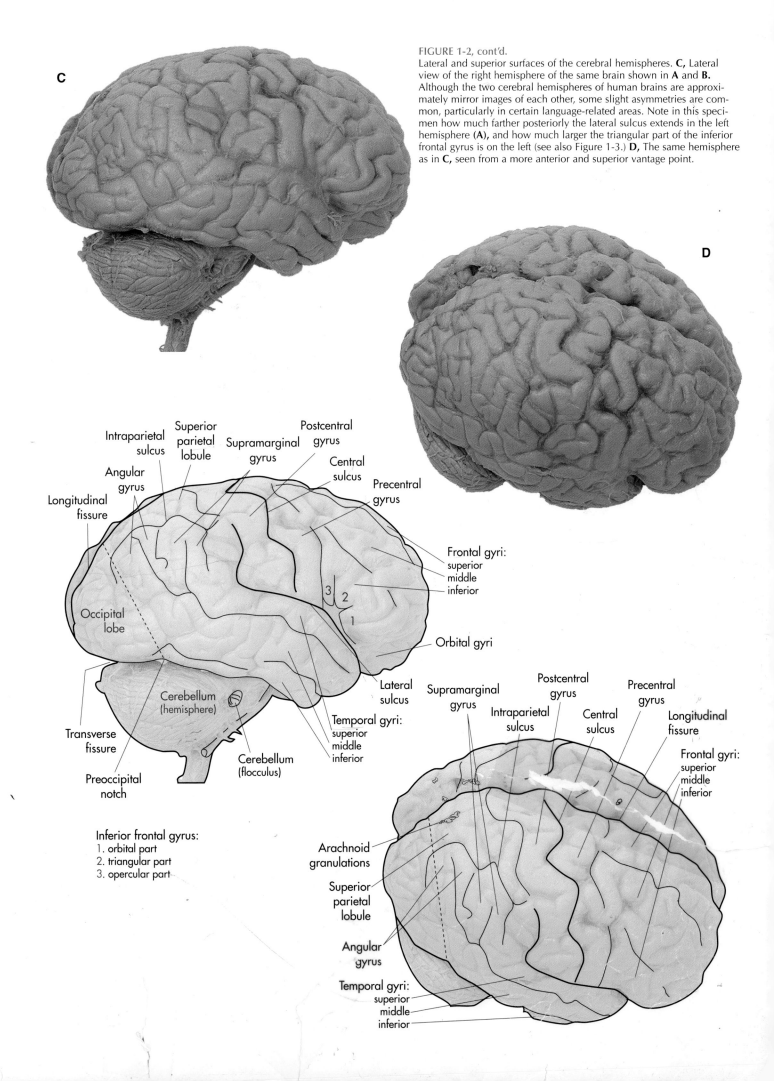

FIGURE 1-2, cont'd.
Lateral and superior surfaces of the cerebral hemispheres. **C,** Lateral view of the right hemisphere of the same brain shown in **A** and **B.** Although the two cerebral hemispheres of human brains are approximately mirror images of each other, some slight asymmetries are common, particularly in certain language-related areas. Note in this specimen how much farther posteriorly the lateral sulcus extends in the left hemisphere **(A),** and how much larger the triangular part of the inferior frontal gyrus is on the left (see also Figure 1-3.) **D,** The same hemisphere as in **C,** seen from a more anterior and superior vantage point.

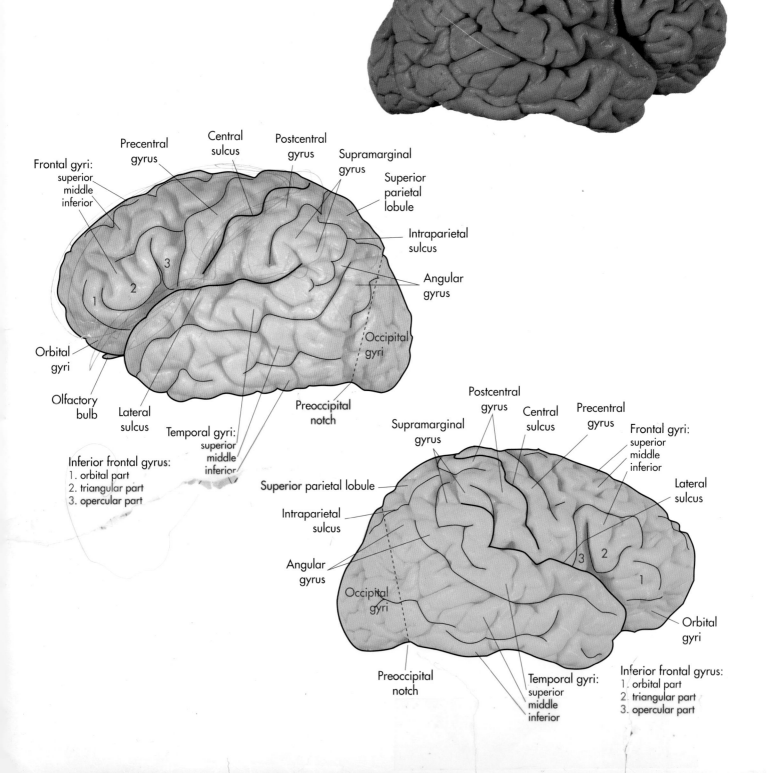

FIGURE 1-3
A and **B,** The left and right cerebral hemispheres of the brain shown in Figures 1-1, *A* and 1-6, shown at about half actual size. Note in this specimen how much farther posteriorly the lateral sulcus extends in the left hemisphere **(A),** and how much larger the triangular and opercular parts of the inferior frontal gyrus are on the left. **A,** Lateral view of the left hemisphere. **B,** Lateral view of the right hemisphere. *(Dissections courtesy of Grant Dahmer, Department of Cell Biology and Anatomy, University of Arizona College of Medicine.)*

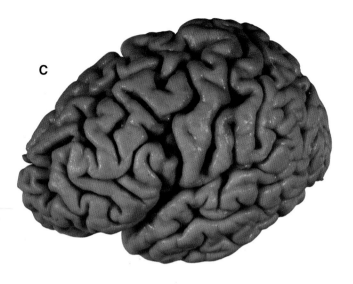

C

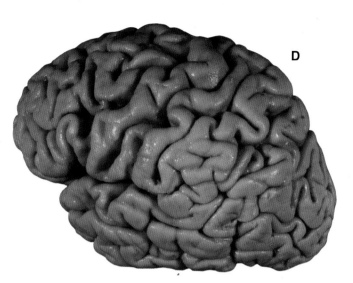

D

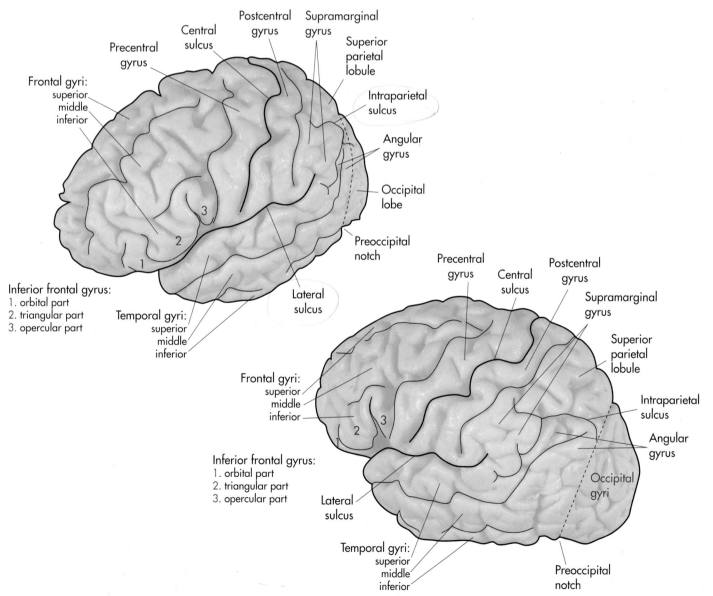

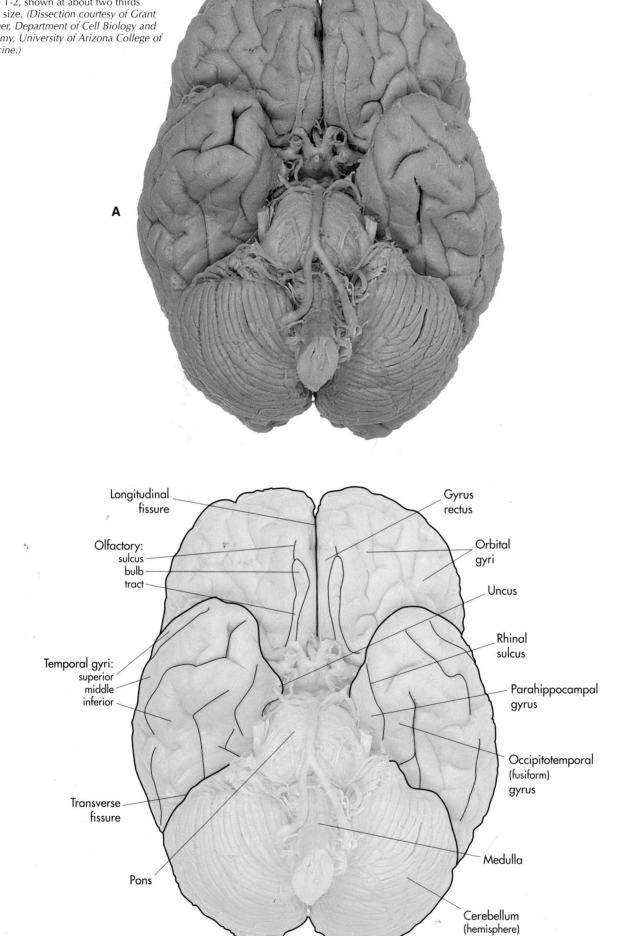

FIGURE 1-4
A, Inferior surface of the same brain as in Figure 1-2, shown at about two thirds actual size. *(Dissection courtesy of Grant Dahmer, Department of Cell Biology and Anatomy, University of Arizona College of Medicine.)*

FIGURE 1-5, cont'd.
B, The diencephalon and part of the brainstem, shown at about 1.7×
actual size.

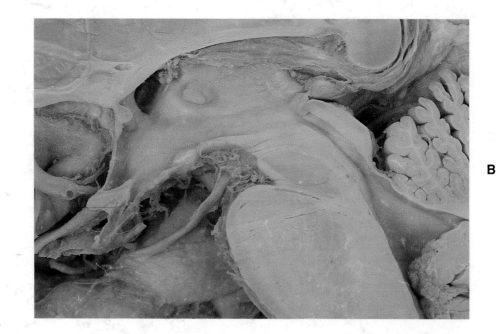

B

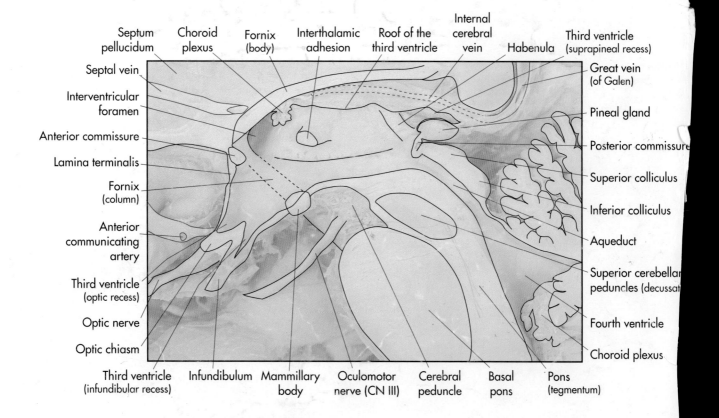

Septum pellucidum
Choroid plexus
Fornix (body)
Interthalamic adhesion
Roof of the third ventricle
Internal cerebral vein
Habenula
Third ventricle (suprapineal recess)

Septal vein
Interventricular foramen
Anterior commissure
Lamina terminalis
Fornix (column)
Anterior communicating artery
Third ventricle (optic recess)
Optic nerve
Optic chiasm

Great vein (of Galen)
Pineal gland
Posterior commissure
Superior colliculus
Inferior colliculus
Aqueduct
Superior cerebellar peduncles (decussat
Fourth ventricle
Choroid plexus

Third ventricle (infundibular recess)
Infundibulum
Mammillary body
Oculomotor nerve (CN III)
Cerebral peduncle
Basal pons
Pons (tegmentum)

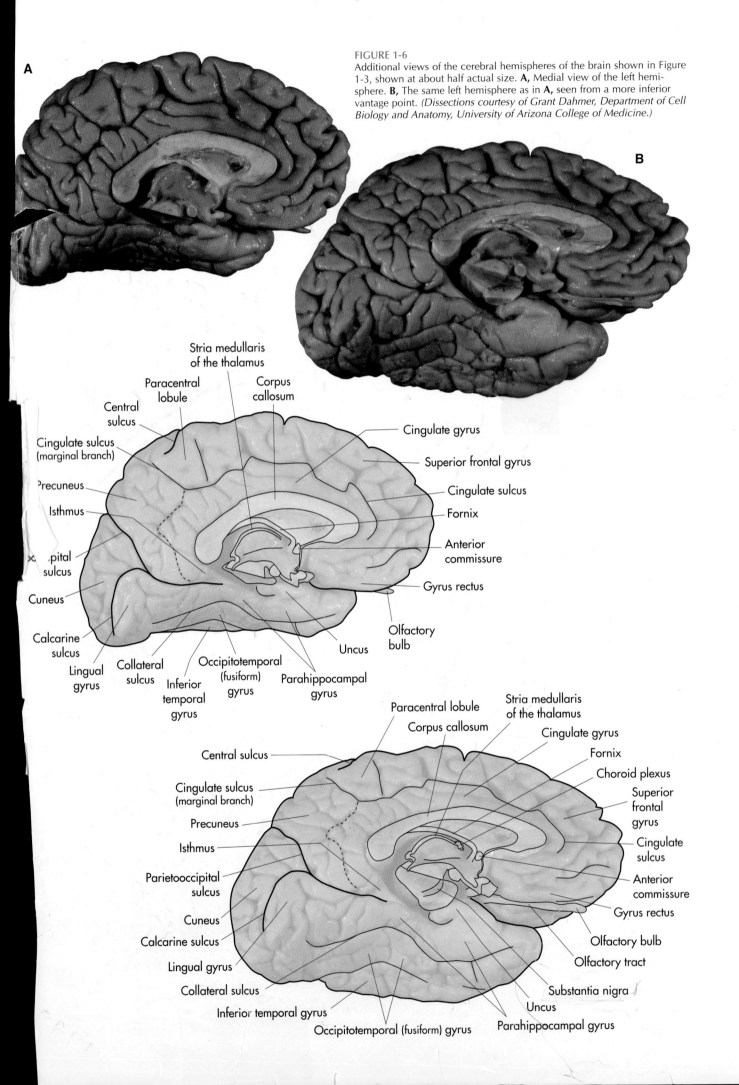

A

B

FIGURE 1-6
Additional views of the cerebral hemispheres of the brain shown in Figure 1-3, shown at about half actual size. **A,** Medial view of the left hemisphere. **B,** The same left hemisphere as in **A,** seen from a more inferior vantage point. *(Dissections courtesy of Grant Dahmer, Department of Cell Biology and Anatomy, University of Arizona College of Medicine.)*

Stria medullaris of the thalamus
Paracentral lobule
Corpus callosum
Central sulcus
Cingulate sulcus (marginal branch)
Precuneus
Isthmus
Occipital sulcus
Cuneus
Calcarine sulcus
Lingual gyrus
Collateral sulcus
Inferior temporal gyrus
Occipitotemporal (fusiform) gyrus
Parahippocampal gyrus
Cingulate gyrus
Superior frontal gyrus
Cingulate sulcus
Fornix
Anterior commissure
Gyrus rectus
Olfactory bulb
Uncus

Paracentral lobule
Corpus callosum
Central sulcus
Cingulate sulcus (marginal branch)
Precuneus
Isthmus
Parietooccipital sulcus
Cuneus
Calcarine sulcus
Lingual gyrus
Collateral sulcus
Inferior temporal gyrus
Occipitotemporal (fusiform) gyrus
Parahippocampal gyrus
Stria medullaris of the thalamus
Cingulate gyrus
Fornix
Choroid plexus
Superior frontal gyrus
Cingulate sulcus
Anterior commissure
Gyrus rectus
Olfactory bulb
Olfactory tract
Substantia nigra
Uncus

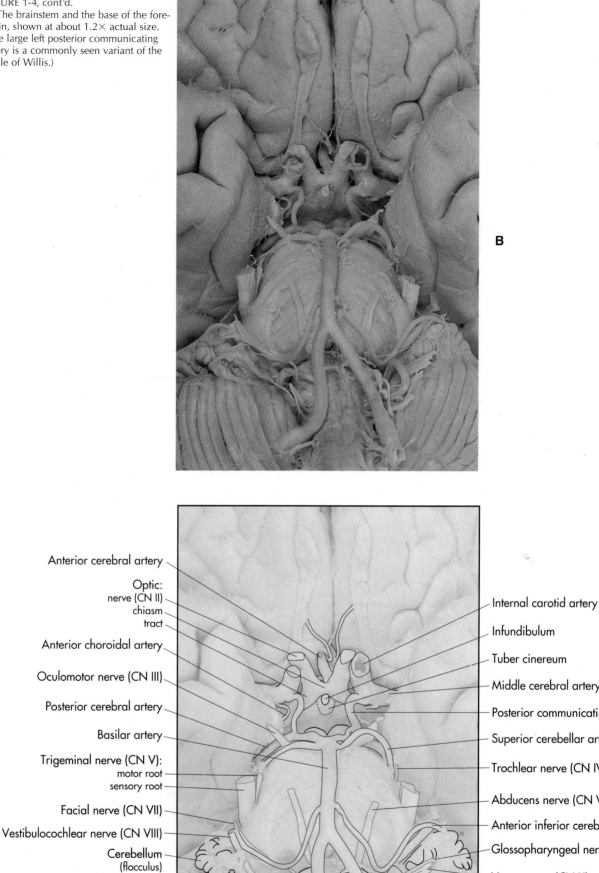

FIGURE 1-4, cont'd.
B, The brainstem and the base of the fore-brain, shown at about 1.2× actual size. (The large left posterior communicating artery is a commonly seen variant of the circle of Willis.)

B

Anterior cerebral artery

Optic:
nerve (CN II)
chiasm
tract

Anterior choroidal artery

Oculomotor nerve (CN III)

Posterior cerebral artery

Basilar artery

Trigeminal nerve (CN V):
motor root
sensory root

Facial nerve (CN VII)

Vestibulocochlear nerve (CN VIII)

Cerebellum
(flocculus)

Choroid plexus
(in lateral aperture)

Posterior inferior cerebellar artery

Anterior spinal artery

Vertebral artery

Internal carotid artery

Infundibulum

Tuber cinereum

Middle cerebral artery

Posterior communicating artery

Superior cerebellar artery

Trochlear nerve (CN IV)

Abducens nerve (CN VI)

Anterior inferior cerebellar artery

Glossopharyngeal nerve (CN IX)

Vagus nerve (CN X)

Hypoglossal nerve (CN XII)

Cervical ventral root (C1)

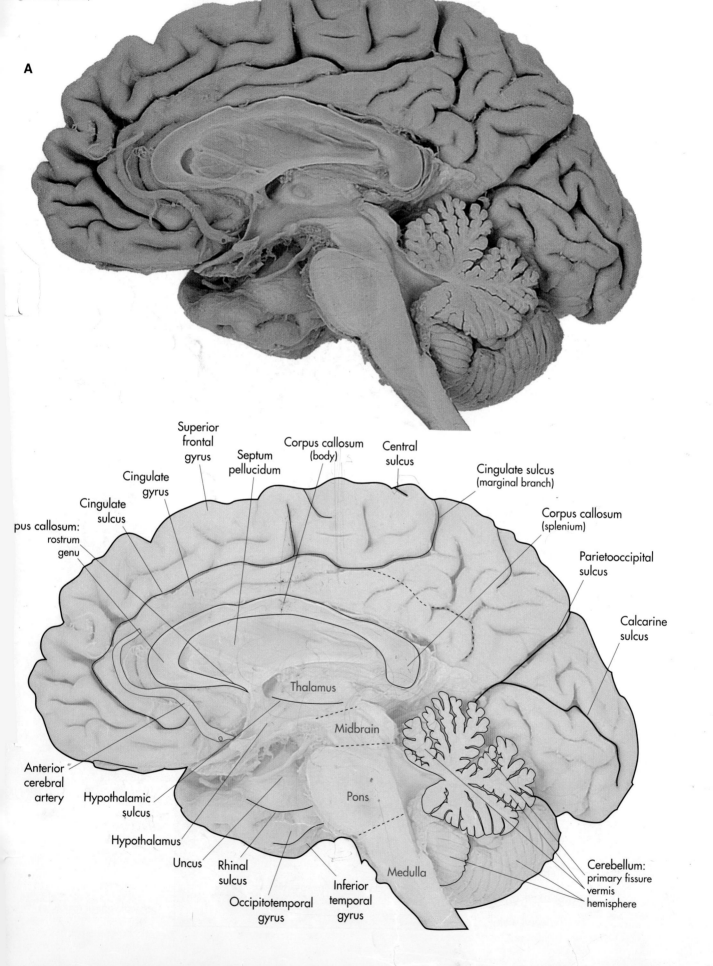

Medial surface of the right half of a sagittally hemisected brain, shown actual size. (Dissection courtesy of Grant Dahmer, Department f Cell Biology and Anatomy, University of Arizona 'ollege of Medicine.)

A

Superior
frontal
gyrus

Septum
pellucidum

Corpus callosum
(body)

Central
sulcus

Cingulate
gyrus

Cingulate sulcus
(marginal branch)

Cingulate
sulcus

Corpus callosum
(splenium)

pus callosum:
rostrum
genu

Parietooccipital
sulcus

Calcarine
sulcus

Thalamus

Midbrain

Pons

Anterior
cerebral
artery

Hypothalamic
sulcus

Medulla

Cerebellum:
primary fissure
vermis
hemisphere

Hypothalamus

Uncus

Rhinal
sulcus

Occipitotemporal
gyrus

Inferior
temporal
gyrus

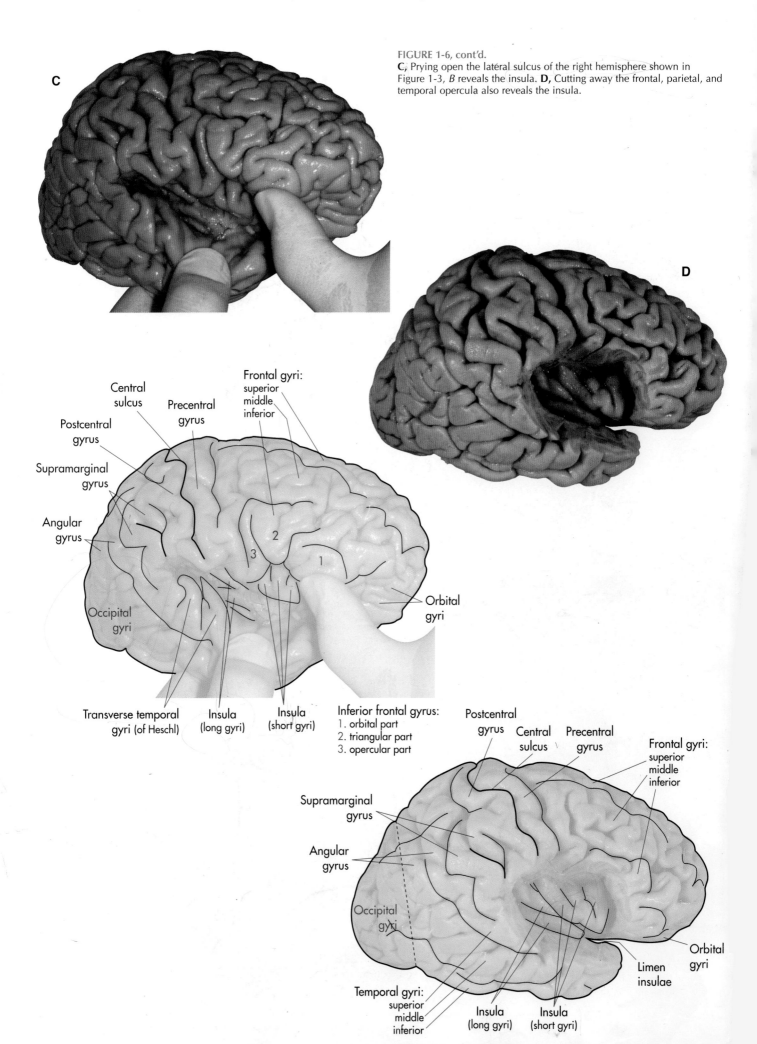

C

D

FIGURE 1-6, cont'd.
C, Prying open the lateral sulcus of the right hemisphere shown in Figure 1-3, *B* reveals the insula. **D,** Cutting away the frontal, parietal, and temporal opercula also reveals the insula.

Central sulcus

Precentral gyrus

Postcentral gyrus

Frontal gyri:
superior
middle
inferior

Supramarginal gyrus

Angular gyrus

Occipital gyri

Orbital gyri

Transverse temporal gyri (of Heschl)

Insula (long gyri)

Insula (short gyri)

Inferior frontal gyrus:
1. orbital part
2. triangular part
3. opercular part

Postcentral gyrus

Central sulcus

Precentral gyrus

Frontal gyri:
superior
middle
inferior

Supramarginal gyrus

Angular gyrus

Occipital gyri

Orbital gyri

Limen insulae

Temporal gyri:
superior
middle
inferior

Insula (long gyri)

Insula (short gyri)

FIGURE 1-7
Inferior and lateral views of the cerebrum and brainstem, demonstrating the cranial nerves. **A,** Inferior view, shown at about two thirds actual size. **B,** Lateral and inferior view, shown at about 2.7× actual size. *(Dissection courtesy of Dr. Norman Koelling, Department of Cell Biology and Anatomy, University of Arizona College of Medicine.)*

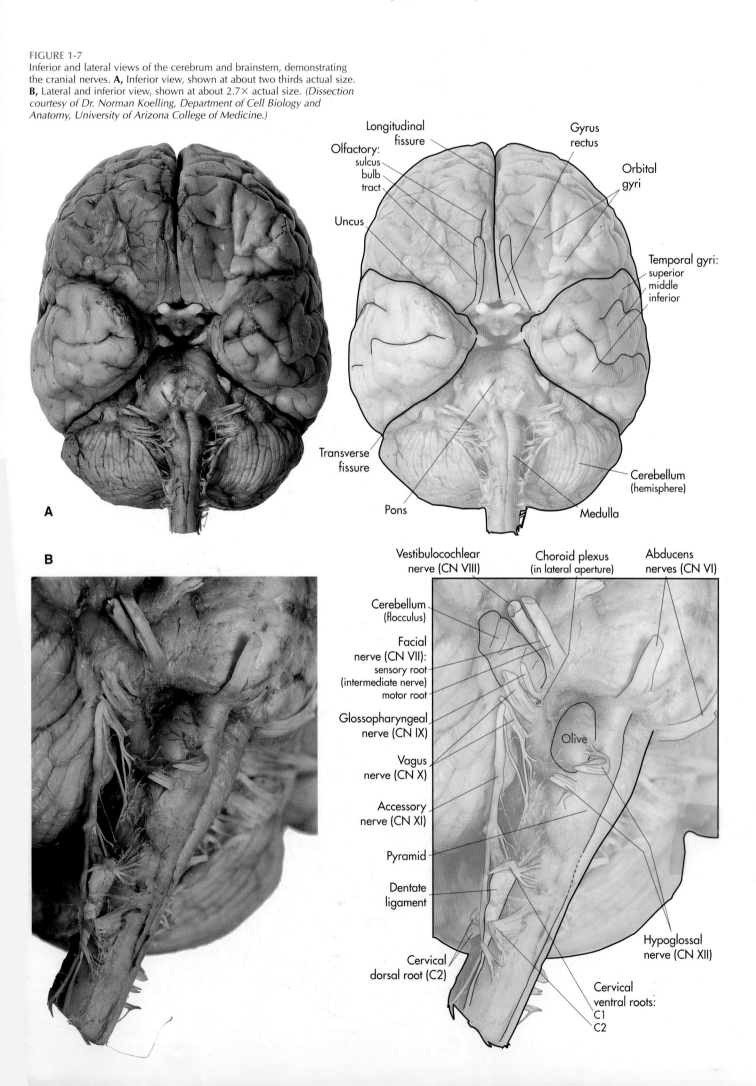

FIGURE 1-7, cont'd.
C, Inferior view, shown at about 1.4×
actual size.

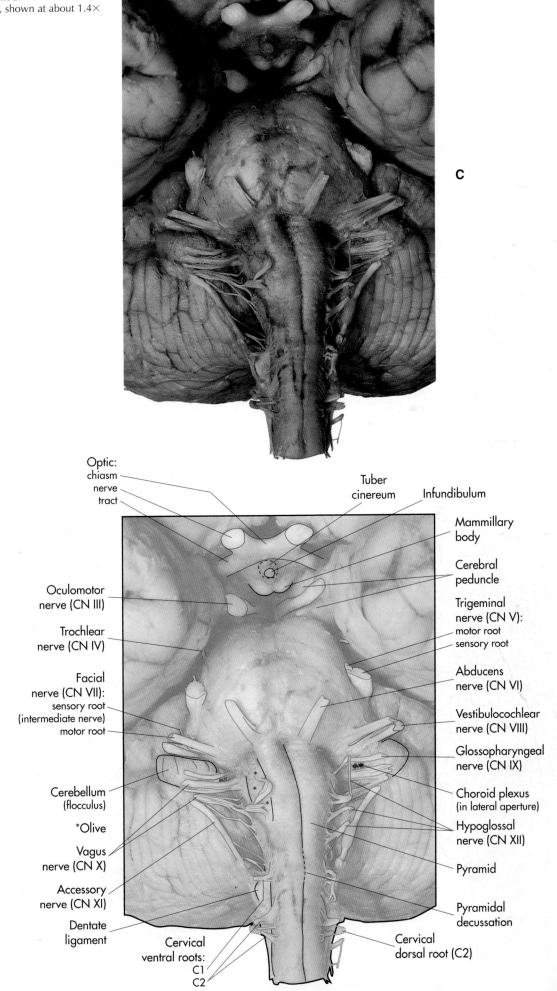

C

Optic:
chiasm
nerve
tract

Tuber
cinereum

Infundibulum

Mammillary
body

Cerebral
peduncle

Oculomotor
nerve (CN III)

Trochlear
nerve (CN IV)

Trigeminal
nerve (CN V):
motor root
sensory root

Facial
nerve (CN VII):
sensory root
(intermediate nerve)
motor root

Abducens
nerve (CN VI)

Vestibulocochlear
nerve (CN VIII)

Glossopharyngeal
nerve (CN IX)

Cerebellum
(flocculus)

Choroid plexus
(in lateral aperture)

*Olive

Hypoglossal
nerve (CN XII)

Vagus
nerve (CN X)

Pyramid

Accessory
nerve (CN XI)

Pyramidal
decussation

Dentate
ligament

Cervical
ventral roots:
C1
C2

Cervical
dorsal root (C2)

FIGURE 1-8
Four views of a brainstem, shown at about 1.3× actual size. *(Dissection courtesy of Grant Dahmer, Department of Anatomy, The University of Arizona College of Medicine.)*

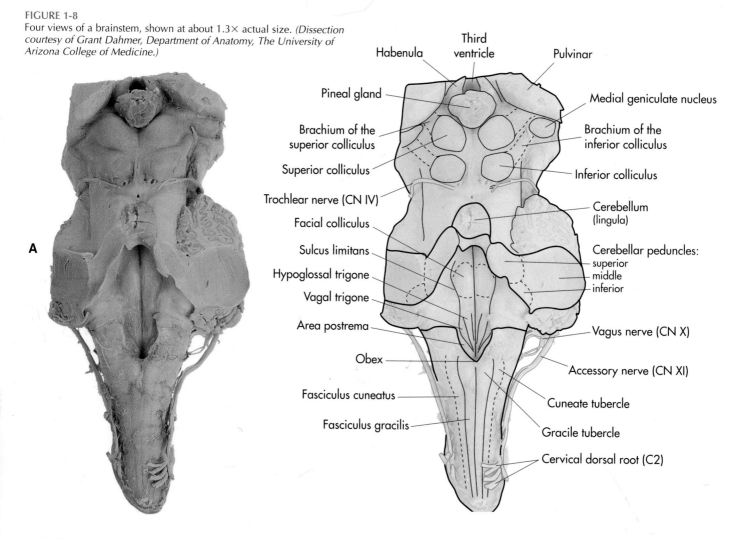

A, The dorsal surface, looking down on the floor of the fourth ventricle.

B, The ventral surface.

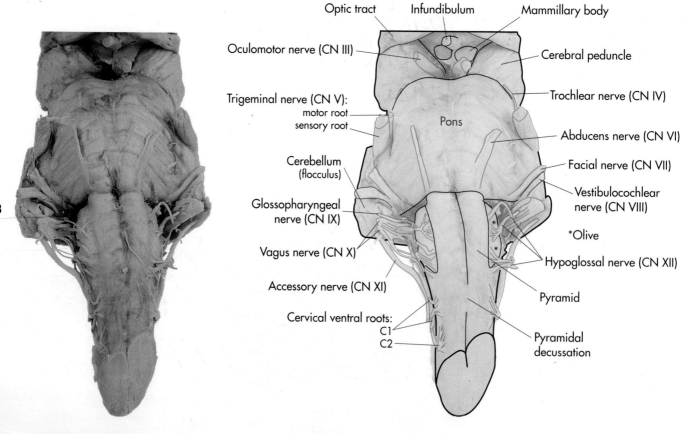

FIGURE 1-8, cont'd.
Four views of a brainstem. **C,** Right side. **D,** Left side.

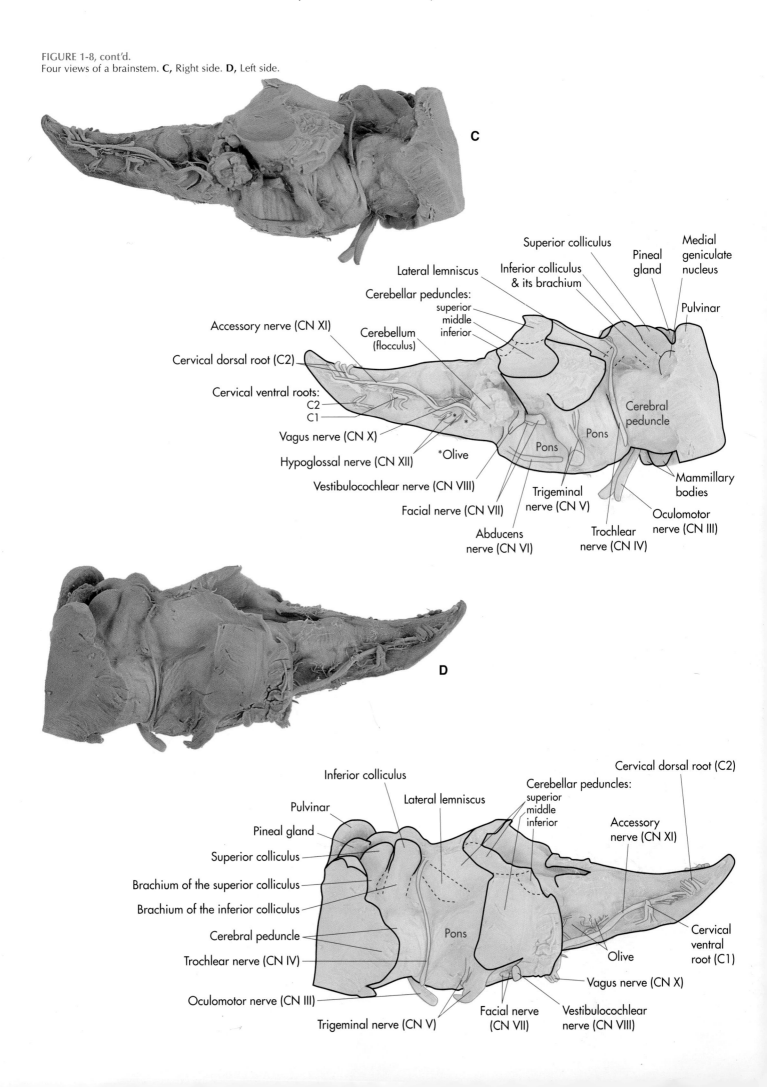

C

Superior colliculus
Lateral lemniscus
Inferior colliculus
& its brachium
Cerebellar peduncles:
superior
middle
inferior
Pineal
gland
Medial
geniculate
nucleus
Pulvinar
Accessory nerve (CN XI)
Cerebellum
(flocculus)
Cervical dorsal root (C2)
Cervical ventral roots:
C2
C1
Vagus nerve (CN X)
Hypoglossal nerve (CN XII)
Vestibulocochlear nerve (CN VIII)
Facial nerve (CN VII)
Abducens
nerve (CN VI)
*Olive
Trigeminal
nerve (CN V)
Pons
Pons
Pons
Cerebral
peduncle
Mammillary
bodies
Oculomotor
nerve (CN III)
Trochlear
nerve (CN IV)

D

Inferior colliculus
Pulvinar
Lateral lemniscus
Pineal gland
Superior colliculus
Brachium of the superior colliculus
Brachium of the inferior colliculus
Cerebral peduncle
Trochlear nerve (CN IV)
Oculomotor nerve (CN III)
Trigeminal nerve (CN V)
Cerebellar peduncles:
superior
middle
inferior
Cervical dorsal root (C2)
Accessory
nerve (CN XI)
Cervical
ventral
root (C1)
Olive
Vagus nerve (CN X)
Facial nerve
(CN VII)
Vestibulocochlear
nerve (CN VIII)
Pons

TRANSVERSE SECTIONS OF THE SPINAL CORD

The spinal cord is perhaps the most simply arranged part of the CNS. Its basic structure, indicated in a schematic drawing of the eighth cervical segment (Figure 2-1), is the same at every level—a butterfly-shaped core of gray matter surrounded by white matter. An often indistinct central canal in the middle of the butterfly is the remnant of the lumen of the embryonic neural tube.

The extensions of the gray matter posteriorly and anteriorly are termed the posterior and anterior (dorsal and ventral) horns, respectively. The zone where the two horns meet is the intermediate gray. At every level, the posterior horn is capped by a zone of closely packed small neurons, the substantia gelatinosa. Beyond this, there are level-to-level variations in the configuration of the spinal gray (Figure 2-2). For example, the motor neurons that innervate skeletal muscle are located in the anterior horns, so these horns expand laterally in lumbar and lower cervical segments to accommodate the many motor neurons required for the muscles of the lower and upper extremities. Other examples are pointed out in Figure 2-2. When studied in detail, the spinal gray matter can be partitioned into a series of 10 layers (Rexed's laminae), as indicated on the right side of Figure 2-1. Some of these laminae have clear functional significance. For example, lamina II corresponds to the substantia gelatinosa, which plays an important role in regulating painful and thermal sensations.

Spinal white matter contains pathways ascending to or descending from higher levels of the nervous system, as well as nerve fibers interconnecting different levels of the spinal cord.

The horns of the gray matter serve to divide the white matter into posterior, lateral, and anterior funiculi. In contrast to the level-to-level variations in the gray matter, the total amount of white matter increases steadily at progressively higher spinal levels. Moving rostrally, the ascending pathways enlarge as progressively more fibers are added to them; the descending pathways do the same because fewer fibers have left them.

Information travels to and from the spinal gray matter in the dorsal and ventral roots. The dorsal roots convey the central processes of afferents with cell bodies in dorsal root ganglia. As the roots approach the spinal cord they break up into filaments, each of which sorts itself into a medial division, containing the large-diameter afferents, and a lateral division, containing the small-diameter afferents. This is the beginning of two great streams of somatosensory information that travel rostrally in the CNS. The large fibers, primarily carrying information about touch and position, send branches into multiple levels of the gray matter and may send a branch rostrally in the posterior funiculus. The small fibers, primarily carrying information about pain and temperature, traverse a distinctive area of the white matter (Lissauer's tract) and end more superficially in the posterior horn. Subsequent connections of both classes of afferents are reviewed in Chapter 8.

In the pages that follow (as in all chapters in this atlas), only the largest and best known spinal structures and pathways are indicated. Many others are either known to exist in humans or inferred from animal studies. In many cases, however, their functional significance is not well understood.

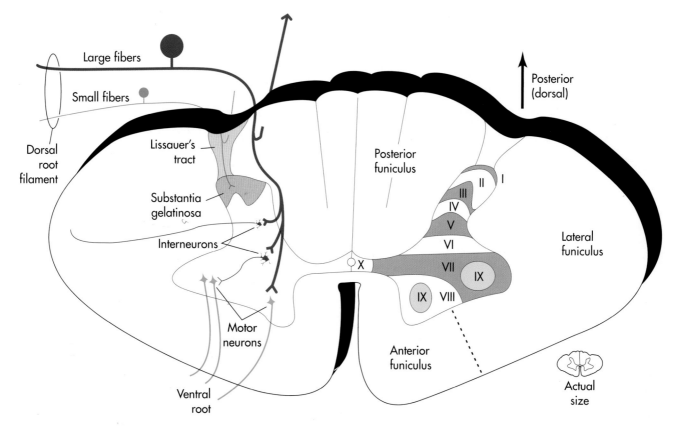

FIGURE 2-1
Schematic drawing of the spinal cord at the level of the eighth cervical segment. *(Modified from Nolte J: The human brain, ed 4, St. Louis, 1999, Mosby.)*

FIGURE 2-2
Cross sections of a spinal cord at eight different levels.

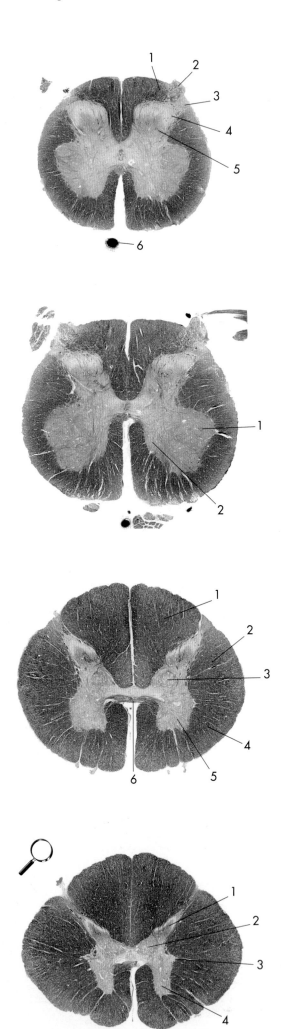

A, The fourth sacral segment (S4). Several features common to all spinal levels can be seen. The substantia gelatinosa *(4)* caps the posterior horn *(5)*. Also, afferent fibers entering through dorsal rootlets *(2)* sort themselves into small-diameter fibers that move laterally and enter Lissauer's tract *(3)* and large-diameter fibers that enter more medially *(1)* at the edge of the posterior funiculus. (This sorting occurs at all spinal levels and can be seen in all of the sections in this series.) Little white matter is present in any of the funiculi because most fibers have either already left descending pathways or not yet entered ascending pathways. The anterior spinal artery *(6)* is cut in cross section as it runs longitudinally near the anterior median fissure of the cord.

B, The fifth lumbar segment (L5). This segment is in the lumbar enlargement (which extends from about L2 to S3) and has anterior horns that are enlarged, primarily in their lateral aspects *(1)*, to accommodate motor neurons for leg and foot muscles. Motor neurons located more medially *(2)* in the anterior horn innervate more proximal muscles, in this case hip muscles.

C, The second lumbar segment (L2). The posterior funiculus *(1)* is larger because ascending fibers carrying touch and position information from the lower limb have been added. The lateral funiculus is also larger, reflecting increased numbers of descending fibers in the lateral corticospinal tract *(2)* and ascending fibers in the spinothalamic tract *(4)*. This section is at the rostral end of the lumbar enlargement, so the anterior horn *(5)* no longer is enlarged laterally. Clarke's nucleus *(3)*, which extends from about T1 to L3 and contains the cells of origin of the posterior spinocerebellar tract, makes its appearance. The anterior white commissure *(6)*, a route through which axons can cross the midline, is present at this and all other spinal levels.

D, The tenth thoracic segment (T10). The posterior *(1)* and anterior *(4)* horns are slender, corresponding to the relative dearth of sensory information arriving at this level and the relatively small number of motor neurons needed. Sympathetic preganglionic neurons form a lateral horn *(3)* containing the intermediolateral cell column, a characteristic feature of thoracic segments. Clarke's nucleus *(2)* is still apparent. Shown enlarged in Figure 2-3.

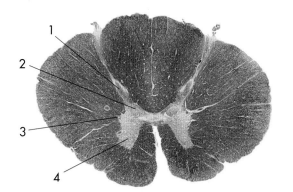

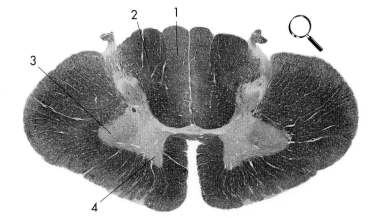

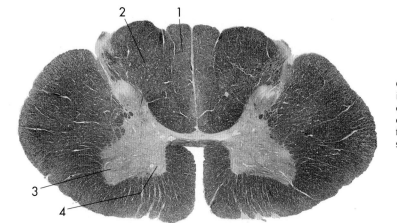

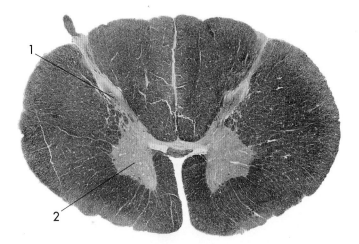

FIGURE 2-2, cont'd.
Cross sections of a spinal cord.

E, The fifth thoracic segment (T5). The posterior *(1)* and anterior *(4)* horns are even more slender, reflecting the relative paucity of sensory information arriving from the trunk and the relatively small number of motor neurons required by trunk muscles. Clarke's nucleus *(2)*, though smaller, is still present, as is the lateral horn *(3)*.

F, The eighth cervical segment (C8), near the caudal end of the cervical enlargement (C5 to T1). The posterior funiculus is subdivided by a partial glial partition into fasciculus gracilis *(1)*, conveying touch and position information from the lower limb, and fasciculus cuneatus *(2)*, conveying touch and position information from the upper limb. The anterior horn is enlarged, primarily in its lateral aspect *(3)*, to accommodate motor neurons for hand and forearm muscles. Motor neurons in more medial parts of the anterior horn *(4)* innervate more proximal muscles, such as the triceps. Shown enlarged in Figure 2-4.

G, The fifth cervical segment (C5), still in the cervical enlargement. As in the previous section, the posterior funiculus is subdivided into fasciculus gracilis *(1)* and fasciculus cuneatus *(2)*, and the anterior horn includes an expanded lateral portion (*3,* here containing motor neurons for forearm muscles) and the more medial area (4) that is present at all spinal levels (and at this level innervates shoulder muscles).

H, The third cervical segment (C3), rostral to the cervical enlargement. The posterior horn *(1)* is more slender, reflecting the smaller amount of afferent input arriving from the neck. The anterior horn *(2)* is no longer enlarged laterally. The area of white matter, however, is larger than in any other section in this series, reflecting the near-maximal size of both ascending and descending pathways.

FIGURE 2-3
Tenth thoracic segment (T10).

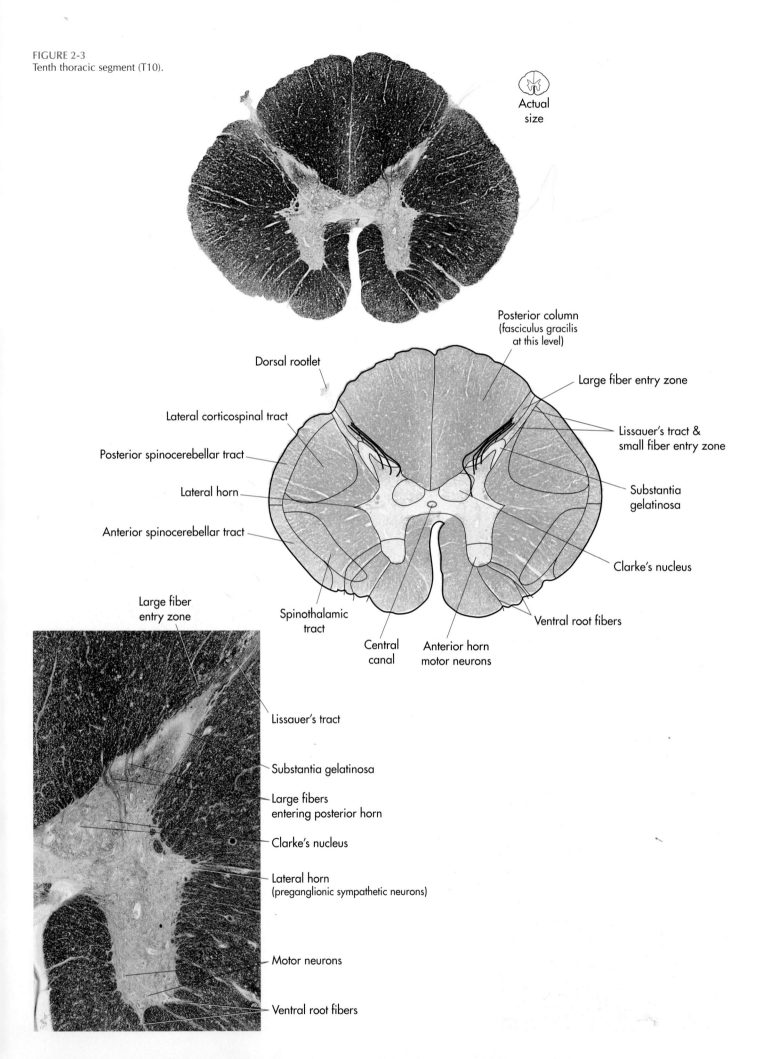

Actual
size

Posterior column
(fasciculus gracilis
at this level)

Dorsal rootlet

Large fiber entry zone

Lateral corticospinal tract

Lissauer's tract &
small fiber entry zone

Posterior spinocerebellar tract

Lateral horn

Substantia
gelatinosa

Anterior spinocerebellar tract

Clarke's nucleus

Ventral root fibers

Large fiber
entry zone

Spinothalamic
tract

Central
canal

Anterior horn
motor neurons

Lissauer's tract

Substantia gelatinosa

Large fibers
entering posterior horn

Clarke's nucleus

Lateral horn
(preganglionic sympathetic neurons)

Motor neurons

Ventral root fibers

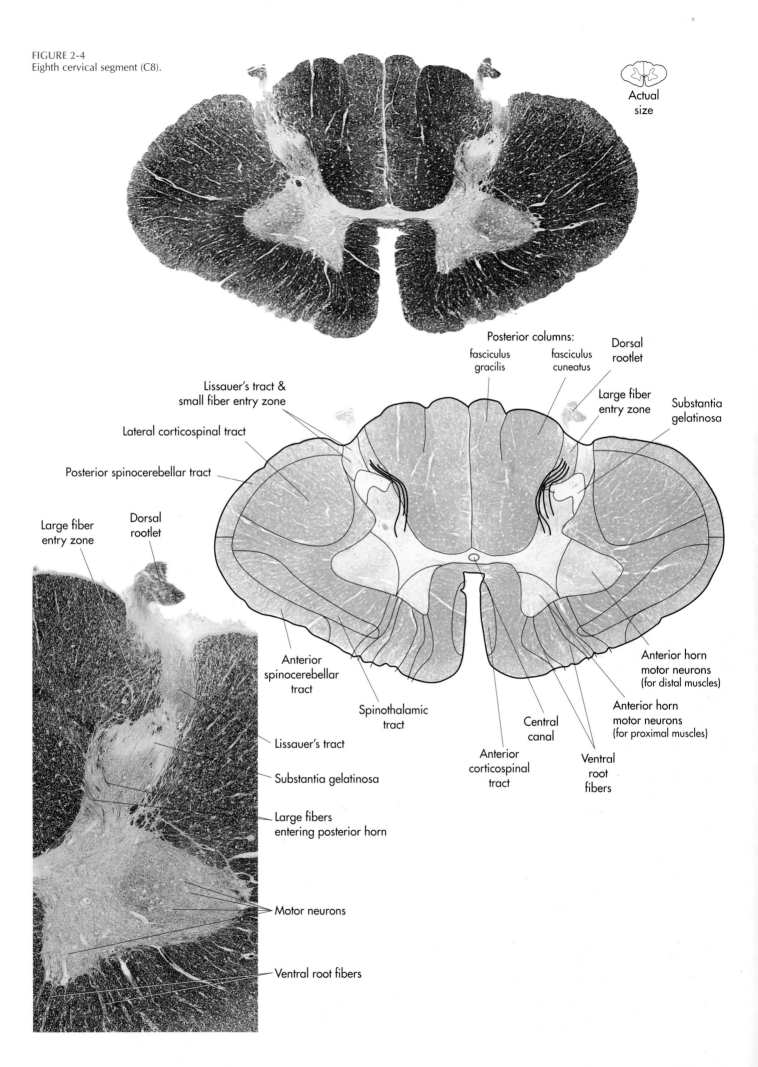

FIGURE 2-4
Eighth cervical segment (C8).

Actual size

Posterior columns:
fasciculus gracilis
fasciculus cuneatus
Dorsal rootlet
Large fiber entry zone
Substantia gelatinosa

Lissauer's tract & small fiber entry zone

Lateral corticospinal tract

Posterior spinocerebellar tract

Large fiber entry zone

Dorsal rootlet

Anterior spinocerebellar tract

Spinothalamic tract

Central canal

Anterior corticospinal tract

Ventral root fibers

Anterior horn motor neurons (for distal muscles)

Anterior horn motor neurons (for proximal muscles)

Lissauer's tract

Substantia gelatinosa

Large fibers entering posterior horn

Motor neurons

Ventral root fibers

FIGURE 3-5
Schematic views of six transverse sections of the brainstem, each enlarged about three times, indicating major long tracts and cranial nerve nuclei. These are the same sections shown photographically in Figures 3-7 to 3-10, 3-12, and 3-13 and they correspond to planes of section indicated in Figure 3-4. Abbreviations as in Figure 3-4.

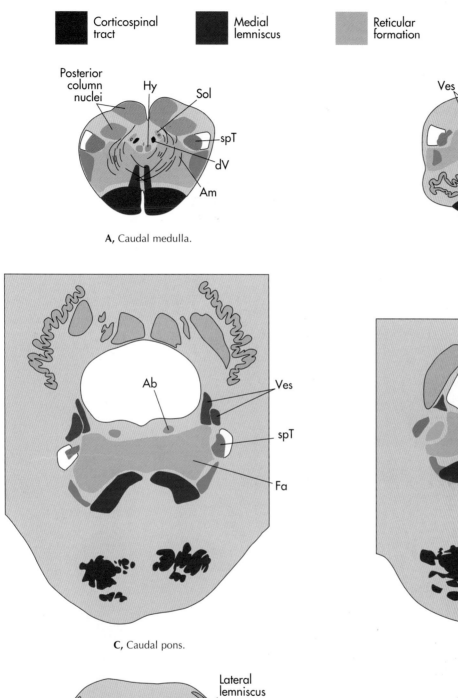

A, Caudal medulla.

B, Rostral medulla.

C, Caudal pons.

D, Midpons.

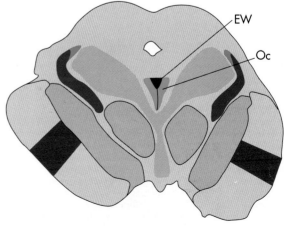

E, Caudal midbrain.

F, Rostral midbrain.

FIGURE 3-6
Cross sections of a brainstem at 12 different levels.

A, Spinomedullary junction. Fasciculus cuneatus *(3)* proceeds rostrally to-ward nucleus cuneatus (not yet present), and fasciculus gracilis *(1)* begins to terminate in nucleus gracilis *(2)*. The spinal trigeminal tract *(4)*, at this level containing trigeminal pain and temperature afferents, and the spinal trigeminal nucleus *(5)* where these afferents terminate, replace Lissauer's tract and the posterior horn of the spinal cord. The spinothalamic tract *(6)* is located ventrolaterally, much as it was in the spinal cord. Corticospinal fibers that descended through the internal capsule, cerebral peduncle, basal pons, and medullary pyramid now cross the midline in the pyrami-dal decussation *(7)*.

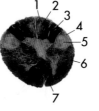

B, Caudal medulla. Fasciculus gracilis has ended in the nucleus gracilis *(1)*, and fasciculus cuneatus *(2)* ends in the nucleus cuneatus *(3)*. Efferents from these posterior column nuclei *(9)* arc across the midline and form the medial lemniscus *(8)*. The spinothalamic tract *(6)* is in its typical loca-tion in the lateral part of the reticular formation, and the corticospinal tract traverses the pyramids *(7)*. Trigeminal primary afferent fibers descend through the spinal trigeminal tract *(4)* to termination sites in the spinal trigeminal nucleus *(5)*. Shown enlarged in Figure 3-7.

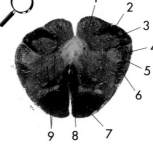

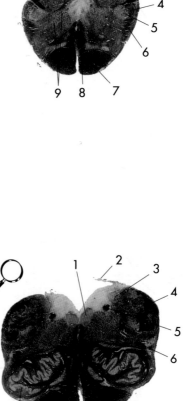

C, Rostral medulla. The central canal of the spinal cord and caudal medulla has given way to the fourth ventricle; part of its roof can be seen *(2)*. Structures associated with cranial nerves appear in the floor of the fourth ventricle, including the hypoglossal nucleus *(1)*, vestibular nuclei *(3)*, and the solitary tract *(5)* surrounded by its nucleus. Efferents from the inferior olivary nucleus *(9)* arc across the midline and join the contralat-eral inferior cerebellar peduncle *(4)*. The locations of the spinothalamic tract *(6)*, medial lemniscus *(8)*, and corticospinal tract *(7)* are unchanged. Shown enlarged in Figure 3-8.

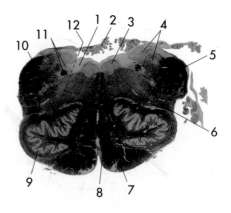

D, Rostral medulla. A plane *(dashed line)* descending from the sulcus lim-itans *(12)* separates cranial nerve nuclei into a more medial group of mo-tor nuclei and a more lateral group of sensory nuclei. Motor nuclei at this level include the hypoglossal nucleus *(3)* and the dorsal motor nucleus of the vagus *(1, adjacent to the sulcus limitans)*. More laterally are the vestibular nuclei *(4)*, spinal trigeminal nucleus *(10)*, and the solitary tract and its nucleus *(11, adjacent to the sulcus limitans)*. The locations of the medial lemniscus *(8)*, spinothalamic tract *(6)*, and corticospinal tract *(7, in the pyramid)* are unchanged. The inferior cerebellar peduncle *(5)* is sub-stantially larger because efferents from the contralateral inferior olivary nucleus *(9)* have accumulated in it. Choroid plexus *(2)* can be seen in the roof of the fourth ventricle.

FIGURE 3-6, cont'd. Cross sections of a brainstem.

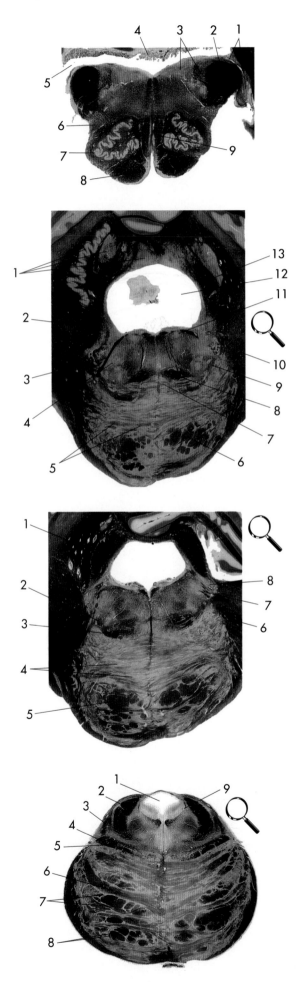

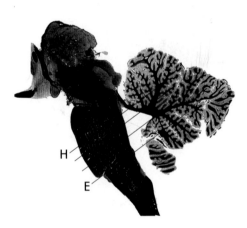

E, Pontomedullary junction. The fourth ventricle extends laterally, leading off into the lateral recess *(5)*; choroid plexus *(4)* is visible in the roof of the ventricle. Vestibular *(3)* and cochlear *(1)* nuclei occupy the ventricular floor. The inferior cerebellar peduncle *(2)* has reached maximum size and is about to enter the cerebellum. The positions of the spinothalamic tract *(6)*, inferior olivary nucleus *(7)*, medial lemniscus *(9)*, and corticospinal tract *(8)* are unchanged.

F, Caudal pons. Now the floor of the fourth ventricle *(12)* is occupied by the abducens nucleus *(11)*, together with facial nerve fibers that emerge from the facial nucleus *(4)*, hook around the abducens nucleus as the genu of the facial nerve, and leave the brainstem as the root of the facial nerve *(3)*. The spinothalamic tract *(9)* is still located laterally in the reticular formation. The medial lemniscus *(8)* begins to move laterally and is traversed by crossing auditory fibers *(7)* of the trapezoid body. The corticospinal tract *(6)* is somewhat dispersed in the basal pons, surrounded by pontine nuclei and their transversely oriented efferents *(5)*, which cross the midline and form the middle cerebellar peduncle *(10)*. Deep cerebellar nuclei *(1)* appear in the roof of the fourth ventricle, and the superior cerebellar peduncle *(13)* begins to form adjacent to them. The inferior cerebellar peduncle *(2)* enters the cerebellum. Shown enlarged in Figure 3-9.

G, Midpons, at the level of entry of the trigeminal nerve *(6)*. Many trigeminal fibers end in the main sensory nucleus of the trigeminal *(8)* or arise in the trigeminal motor nucleus *(7)*. The superior cerebellar peduncle *(1)*, carrying most of the output of the cerebellum, begins to enter the brainstem. The spinothalamic tract *(2)* is still located laterally in the reticular formation, the medial lemniscus *(3)* continues to move laterally, and the corticospinal tract *(5)* is still dispersed in the basal pons *(4)*. Shown enlarged in Figure 3-10.

H, Rostral pons, near the pons–midbrain junction. The fourth ventricle *(1)* narrows as it approaches the aqueduct. The superior cerebellar peduncle *(2)* moves deeper into the brainstem just before beginning to decussate. The medial lemniscus *(5)* is now a flattened band of fibers with the spinothalamic tract *(4)* laterally adjacent to it. The lateral lemniscus *(3)* conveys ascending auditory fibers to the midbrain. The corticospinal tract *(8)* is surrounded by pontine nuclei *(7)* and their transversely oriented efferents *(6)*. The locus ceruleus *(9)* is a small collection of pigmented neurons that provide most of the noradrenergic innervation of the CNS (see Figure 8-33). Shown enlarged in Figure 3-11.

FIGURE 3-6, cont'd. Cross sections of a brainstem.

I, Caudal midbrain. The lateral lemniscus *(4)* ends in the inferior colliculus *(3)*. The spinothalamic tract *(5)* and medial lemniscus *(7)* form a continuous band of fibers. The massive decussation of the superior cerebellar peduncles *(8)* occupies the center of the reticular formation. The basal pons gives way to a cerebral peduncle *(9)* on each side. The tiny trochlear nucleus *(6)* appears. At all midbrain levels the cerebral aqueduct *(1)* is surrounded by periaqueductal gray matter *(2)*. Shown enlarged in Figure 3-12.

J, Mid-midbrain. Characteristic midbrain features such as the aqueduct *(1)* and periaqueductal gray *(2)* can be seen, but no colliculi are present. The brachium of the inferior colliculus *(4)*, spinothalamic tract *(5)*, medial lemniscus *(6)*, and now-crossed superior cerebellar peduncle *(7)* are all on their way to the thalamus. The oculomotor nucleus *(3)*, substantia nigra *(8)*, and cerebral peduncle *(9)* appear—all harbingers of the rostral midbrain.

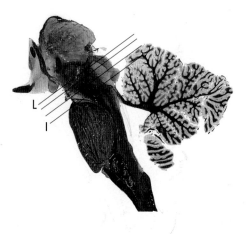

K, Rostral midbrain. Now the superior colliculus *(3)* appears and the oculomotor nucleus *(9)* is fully formed. The auditory pathway continues in the brachium of the inferior colliculus *(4)*. The positions and appearance of the cerebral aqueduct *(1)*, periaqueductal gray *(2)*, spinothalamic tract *(5)*, medial lemniscus *(6)*, and cerebral peduncle *(7)* are little changed. Cerebellar efferents that reached the midbrain in the superior cerebellar peduncle *(10)* now begin to pass through or around the red nucleus. The substantia nigra *(8)* is more prominent. Shown enlarged in Figure 3-13.

L, Rostral midbrain, near the level of the midbrain–diencephalon junction. The cerebral aqueduct *(1)*, periaqueductal gray *(2)*, spinothalamic tract *(3)*, medial lemniscus *(5)*, cerebral peduncle *(6)*, and substantia nigra *(7)* are still evident. The brachium of the inferior colliculus *(4)* ends in the medial geniculate nucleus *(11)*, the first thalamic nucleus to appear in this plane of section. Cerebellar efferents *(9)* pass through and around the red nucleus *(8)* on their way to the thalamus. The ventral tegmental area *(10)* is a medial collection of neurons that provide the dopaminergic innervation of frontal cortex and limbic structures (see Figure 8-34). Efferents from some retinal ganglion cells and visual cortex traverse the brachium of the superior colliculus *(12)* on their way to the superior colliculus.

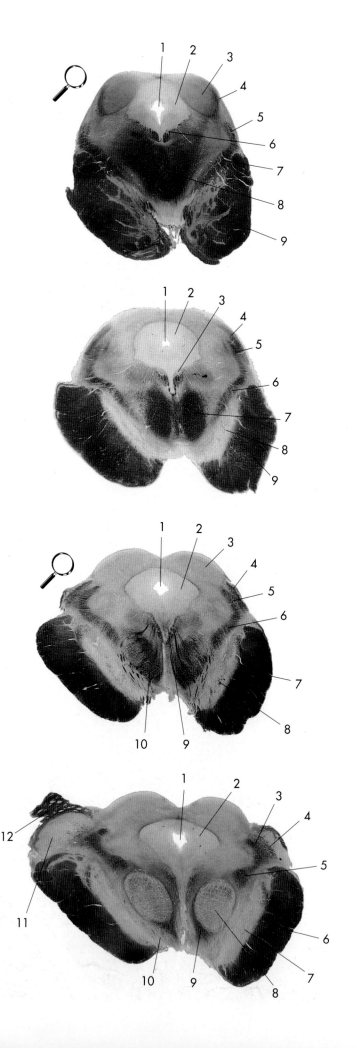

FIGURE 3-7
Caudal medulla.

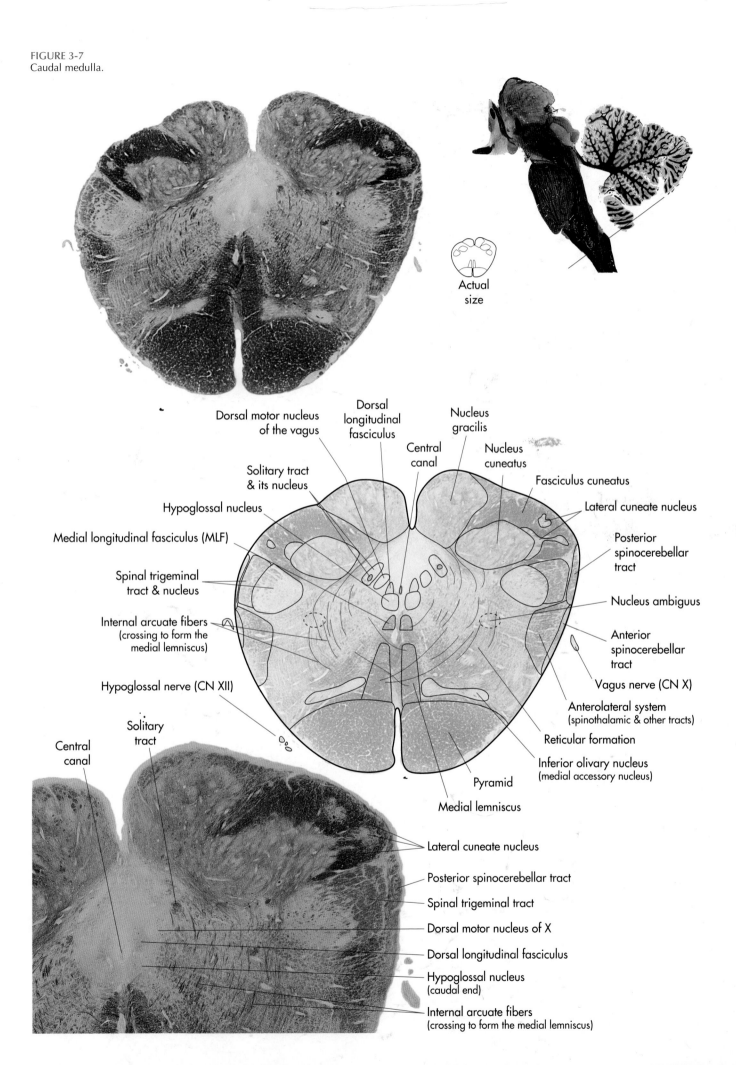

Actual
size

Dorsal motor nucleus
of the vagus

Dorsal
longitudinal
fasciculus

Nucleus
gracilis

Central
canal

Nucleus
cuneatus

Solitary tract
& its nucleus

Fasciculus cuneatus

Hypoglossal nucleus

Lateral cuneate nucleus

Medial longitudinal fasciculus (MLF)

Posterior
spinocerebellar
tract

Spinal trigeminal
tract & nucleus

Nucleus ambiguus

Internal arcuate fibers
(crossing to form the
medial lemniscus)

Anterior
spinocerebellar
tract

Hypoglossal nerve (CN XII)

Vagus nerve (CN X)

Solitary
tract

Anterolateral system
(spinothalamic & other tracts)

Central
canal

Reticular formation

Inferior olivary nucleus
(medial accessory nucleus)

Pyramid

Medial lemniscus

Lateral cuneate nucleus

Posterior spinocerebellar tract

Spinal trigeminal tract

Dorsal motor nucleus of X

Dorsal longitudinal fasciculus

Hypoglossal nucleus
(caudal end)

Internal arcuate fibers
(crossing to form the medial lemniscus)

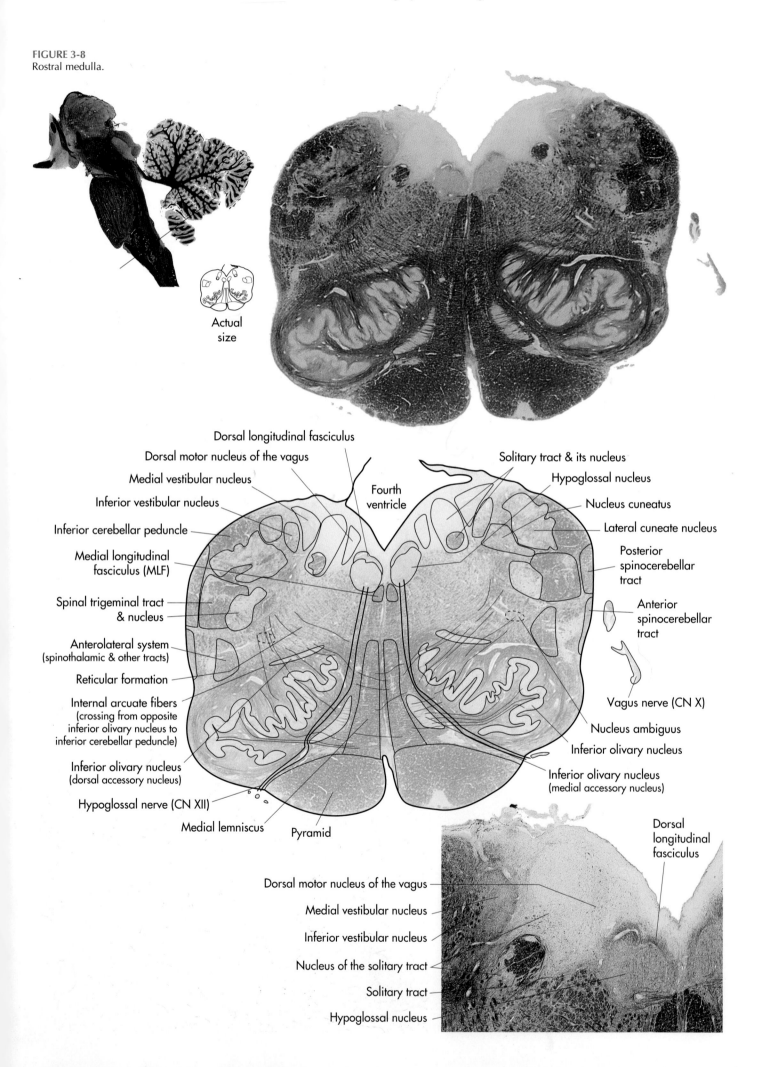

FIGURE 3-8
Rostral medulla.

Actual
size

Dorsal longitudinal fasciculus

Dorsal motor nucleus of the vagus

Medial vestibular nucleus

Inferior vestibular nucleus

Inferior cerebellar peduncle

Medial longitudinal
fasciculus (MLF)

Spinal trigeminal tract
& nucleus

Anterolateral system
(spinothalamic & other tracts)

Reticular formation

Internal arcuate fibers
(crossing from opposite
inferior olivary nucleus to
inferior cerebellar peduncle)

Inferior olivary nucleus
(dorsal accessory nucleus)

Hypoglossal nerve (CN XII)

Medial lemniscus   Pyramid

Fourth
ventricle

Solitary tract & its nucleus

Hypoglossal nucleus

Nucleus cuneatus

Lateral cuneate nucleus

Posterior
spinocerebellar
tract

Anterior
spinocerebellar
tract

Vagus nerve (CN X)

Nucleus ambiguus

Inferior olivary nucleus

Inferior olivary nucleus
(medial accessory nucleus)

Dorsal
longitudinal
fasciculus

Dorsal motor nucleus of the vagus

Medial vestibular nucleus

Inferior vestibular nucleus

Nucleus of the solitary tract

Solitary tract

Hypoglossal nucleus

FIGURE 3-9
Caudal pons.

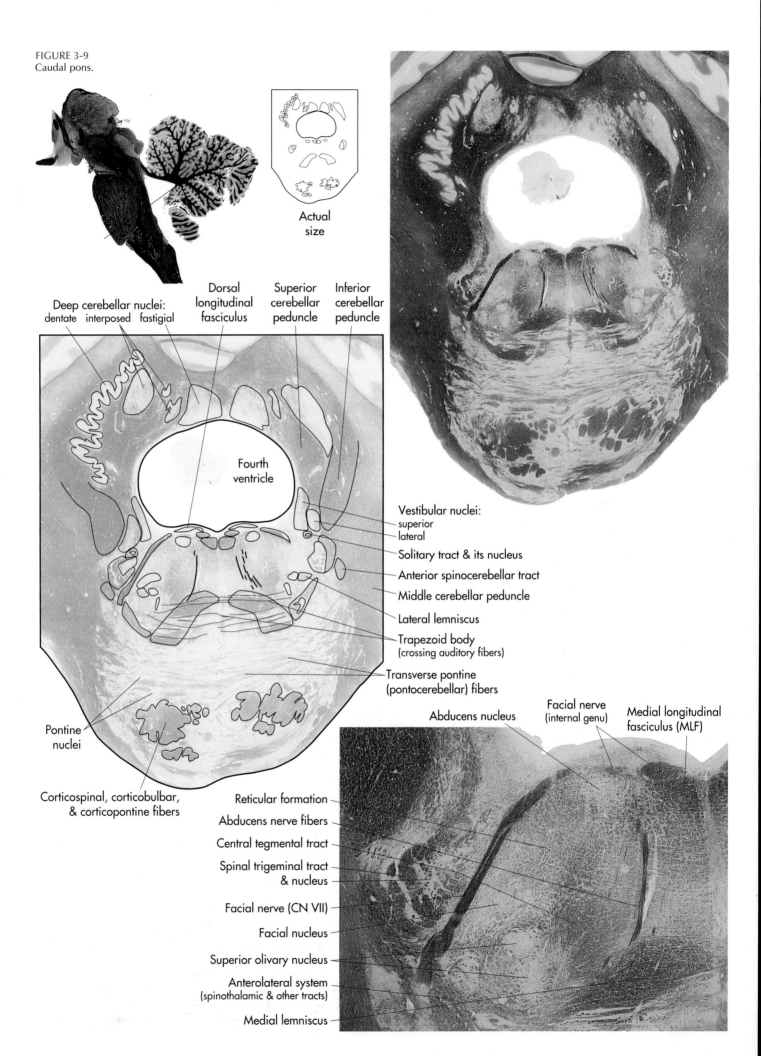

Actual
size

Deep cerebellar nuclei:
dentate   interposed   fastigial

Dorsal
longitudinal
fasciculus

Superior
cerebellar
peduncle

Inferior
cerebellar
peduncle

Fourth
ventricle

Vestibular nuclei:
superior
lateral

Solitary tract & its nucleus

Anterior spinocerebellar tract

Middle cerebellar peduncle

Lateral lemniscus

Trapezoid body
(crossing auditory fibers)

Transverse pontine
(pontocerebellar) fibers

Pontine
nuclei

Corticospinal, corticobulbar,
& corticopontine fibers

Abducens nucleus

Facial nerve
(internal genu)

Medial longitudinal
fasciculus (MLF)

Reticular formation

Abducens nerve fibers

Central tegmental tract

Spinal trigeminal tract
& nucleus

Facial nerve (CN VII)

Facial nucleus

Superior olivary nucleus

Anterolateral system
(spinothalamic & other tracts)

Medial lemniscus

FIGURE 3-10
Midpons.

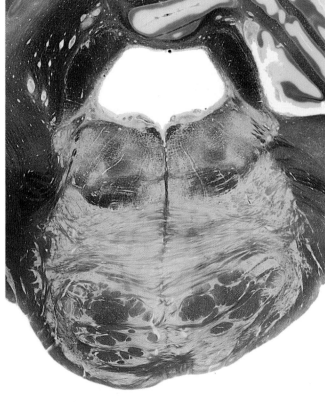

Actual
size

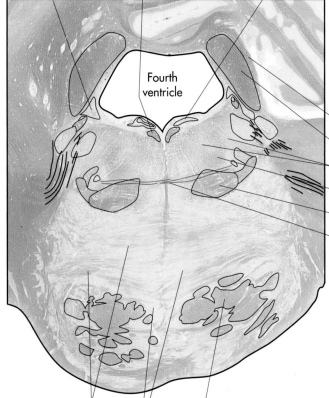

Superior
vestibular
nucleus

Medial longitudinal
fasciculus (MLF)

Dorsal
longitudinal
fasciculus

Fourth
ventricle

Anterior spinocerebellar tract

Superior cerebellar peduncle

Reticular formation

Central tegmental tract

Medial lemniscus

Trapezoid body
(crossing auditory fibers)

Transverse pontine
(pontocerebellar) fibers

Corticospinal, corticobulbar,
& corticopontine fibers

Pontine
nuclei

Cerebellar cortex:
    granular layer
Purkinje cell layer
    molecular layer

Trigeminal nerve

Trigeminal:
mesencephalic nucleus
mesencephalic tract
main sensory nucleus
motor nucleus

Lateral lemniscus

Superior olivary nucleus

Anterolateral system
(spinothalamic & other tracts)

FIGURE 3-11
Rostral pons.

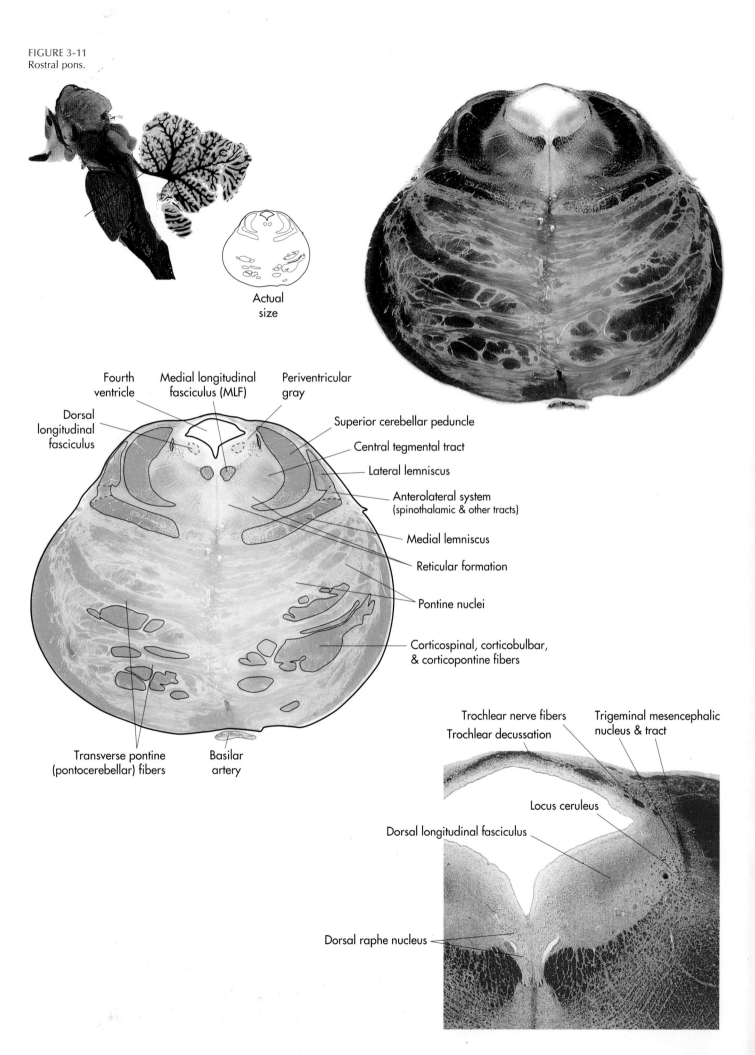

Actual size

Fourth ventricle

Medial longitudinal fasciculus (MLF)

Periventricular gray

Dorsal longitudinal fasciculus

Superior cerebellar peduncle

Central tegmental tract

Lateral lemniscus

Anterolateral system (spinothalamic & other tracts)

Medial lemniscus

Reticular formation

Pontine nuclei

Corticospinal, corticobulbar, & corticopontine fibers

Transverse pontine (pontocerebellar) fibers

Basilar artery

Trochlear nerve fibers
Trochlear decussation

Trigeminal mesencephalic nucleus & tract

Locus ceruleus

Dorsal longitudinal fasciculus

Dorsal raphe nucleus

FIGURE 3-12
Caudal midbrain.

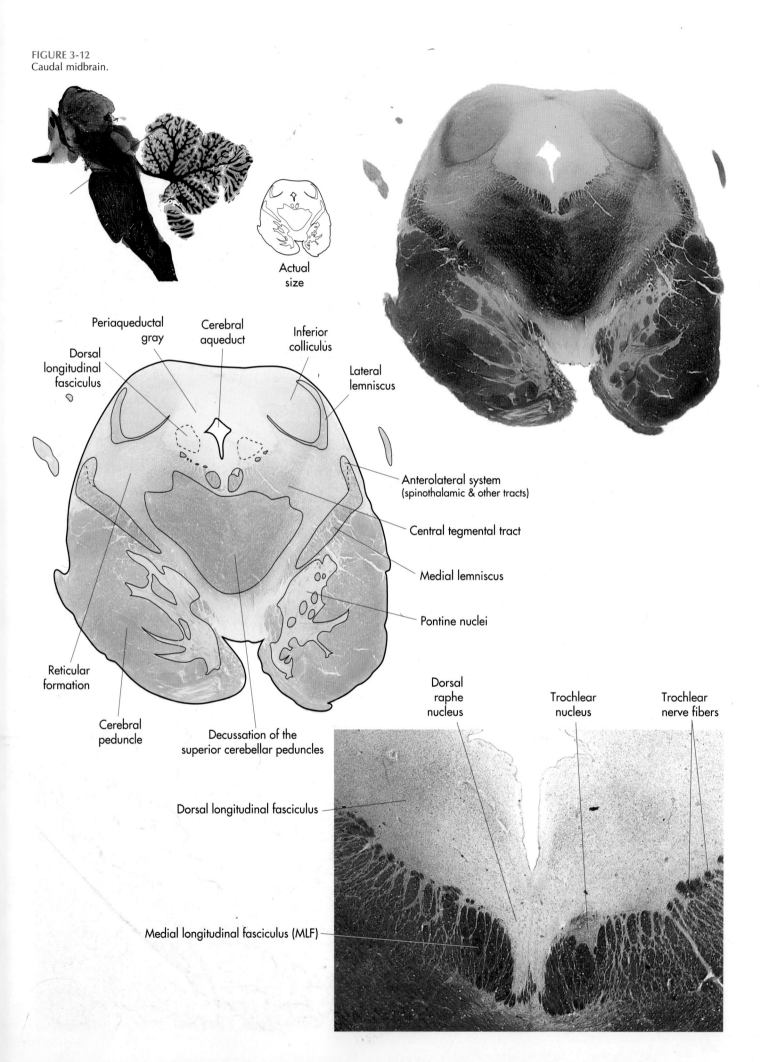

Actual size

Periaqueductal gray

Cerebral aqueduct

Inferior colliculus

Dorsal longitudinal fasciculus

Lateral lemniscus

Anterolateral system (spinothalamic & other tracts)

Central tegmental tract

Medial lemniscus

Pontine nuclei

Reticular formation

Cerebral peduncle

Decussation of the superior cerebellar peduncles

Dorsal raphe nucleus

Trochlear nucleus

Trochlear nerve fibers

Dorsal longitudinal fasciculus

Medial longitudinal fasciculus (MLF)

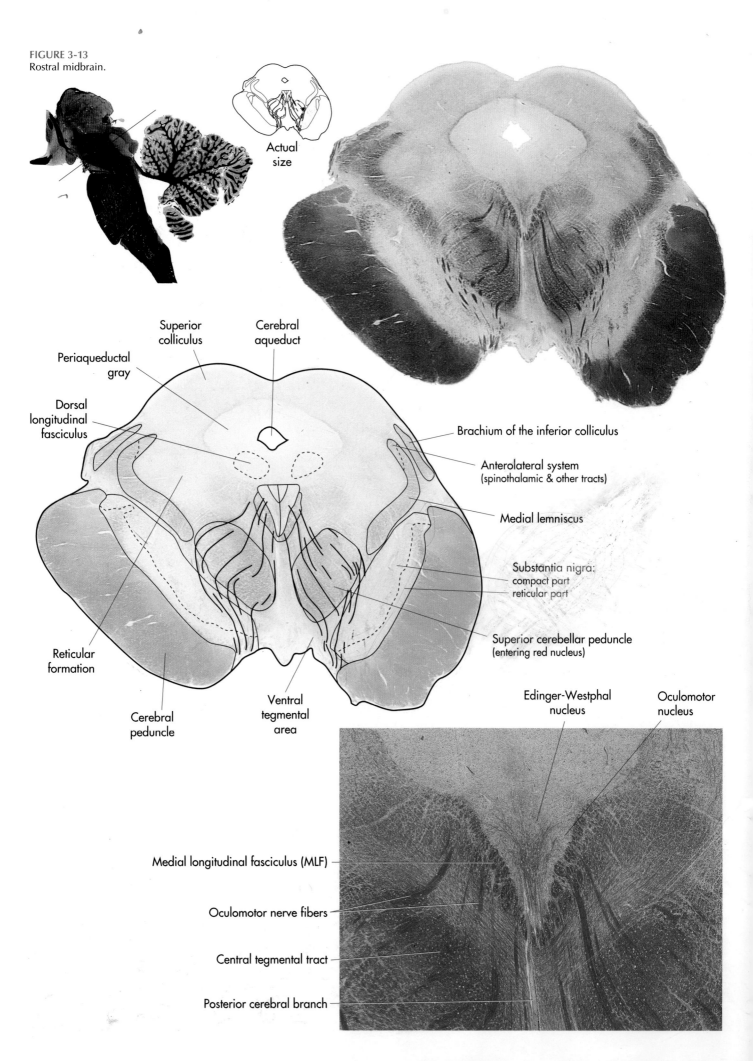

FIGURE 3-13
Rostral midbrain.

Actual size

Superior colliculus

Cerebral aqueduct

Periaqueductal gray

Dorsal longitudinal fasciculus

Brachium of the inferior colliculus

Anterolateral system (spinothalamic & other tracts)

Medial lemniscus

Substantia nigra:
compact part
reticular part

Superior cerebellar peduncle (entering red nucleus)

Reticular formation

Cerebral peduncle

Ventral tegmental area

Edinger-Westphal nucleus

Oculomotor nucleus

Medial longitudinal fasciculus (MLF)

Oculomotor nerve fibers

Central tegmental tract

Posterior cerebral branch

BUILDING A BRAIN:
THREE-DIMENSIONAL RECONSTRUCTIONS

The interior of the cerebrum is occupied by a series of structures that fit neatly together in three-dimensional space. As a consequence of the embryological development of the brain, some cerebral structures (e.g., lateral ventricle, caudate nucleus) curve around in a great C-shaped arch (Figure 4-1), whereas others are more centrally located. One of the greatest impediments to understanding the interrelationships of cerebral structures in three dimensions is the typical presentation of the nervous system in a series of two-dimensional sections cut in various planes (as it is presented in much of this book).

As a partial solution to this dilemma, this chapter presents an overview of the arrangement of cerebral structures in the form of a series of computer-generated reconstructions kindly provided by Dr. John W. Sundsten and his colleagues (Department of Biological Structure, University of Washington School of Medicine). The images were made by cutting serial sections of a single human brain, digitizing outlines of structures of interest, and using these outlines to reconstruct (by computer) individual structures or groups of structures. Beginning with the reconstruction of the brainstem, cerebellum, and diencephalon shown in Figure 4-2, major structures of the cerebral hemispheres are added sequentially in Figure 4-3. Similar three-dimensional reconstructions are used in Chapters 5 through 7 to indicate the planes of sections through the forebrain.

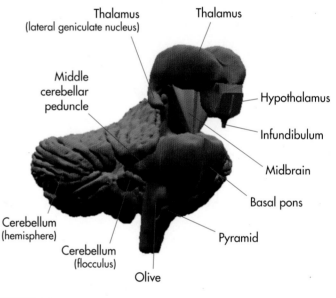

FIGURE 4-2
Three-dimensional reconstruction of the brainstem, cerebellum, and diencephalon. In an intact brain, the hypothalamus is continuous anteriorly with the preoptic and septal areas; in this reconstruction the hypothalamus is shown ending abruptly at its approximate border with these structures. The midbrain is configured with a flattened anterior surface because the cerebral peduncle is not yet present; it will be added in Figure 4-3, *E.*

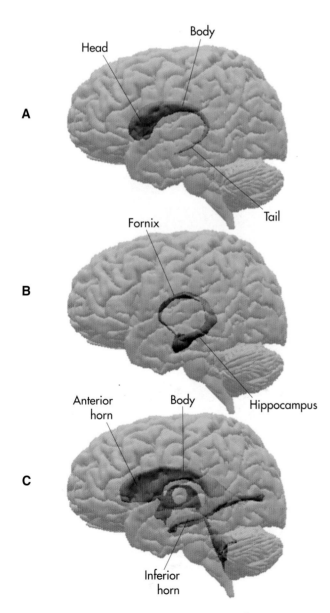

FIGURE 4-1
Three examples of C-shaped telencephalic structures: the caudate nucleus **(A),** hippocampus/fornix system **(B),** and lateral ventricle **(C).** *(Modified from Nolte J: The human brain, ed 4, St. Louis, 1999, Mosby.)*

FIGURE 4-3
Building a brain.

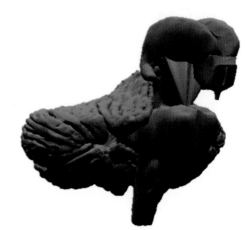

A, The reconstruction of the brainstem, cerebellum, and diencephalon shown in Figure 4-2.

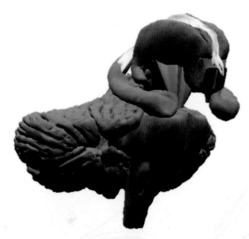

B, The hippocampus *(purple)* is a special cortical area folded into the medial part of the temporal lobe, adjacent to the inferior horn of the lateral ventricle. The fornix *(white)* is a major output pathway from the hippocampus. It curves around in a C-shaped course (the Latin word *fornix* means arch) and terminates primarily in the hypothalamus and septal area.

C, The lateral ventricle is another C-shaped structure, curving from an anterior horn *(1)* in the frontal lobe, through a body *(2),* and into an inferior horn *(5)* in the temporal lobe. A posterior horn *(4)* extends backward into the occipital lobe. The body, posterior horn, and inferior horn meet in the atrium *(3)* of the lateral ventricle. The body and anterior horn have a concave lateral surface; in reality, parts of the caudate nucleus occupy this depression (see Figure 4-3, *D*). The third ventricle *(6)* extends anteriorly beyond the truncated hypothalamus; in an intact brain this anterior extension would be bordered by the preoptic area. The anterior commissure *(7)* contains fibers interconnecting the temporal lobes.

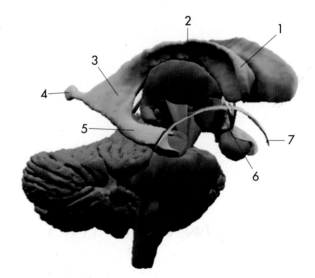

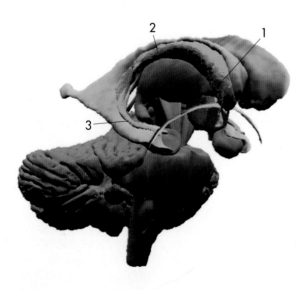

D, The caudate nucleus, yet another C-shaped structure, curves through the hemisphere adjacent to the lateral ventricle. Its enlarged head *(1)* and body *(2)* account for the indented lateral wall of the anterior horn and body of the ventricle (see Figure 4-3, *C*). The attenuated tail *(3)* of the caudate nucleus forms part of the wall of the inferior horn of the ventricle.

FIGURE 4-3, cont'd.
Building a brain.

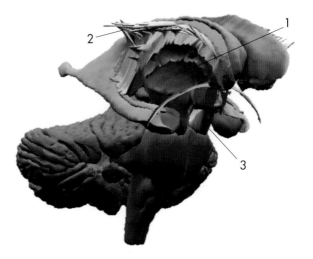

E, The internal capsule *(1)* is a thick band of fibers that covers the lateral aspect of the head of the caudate nucleus and the thalamus. It contains the vast majority of the fibers interconnecting the cerebral cortex and subcortical sites. Above the internal capsule, these fibers fan out within the cerebral hemisphere as the corona radiata *(2).* Many of the cortical efferent fibers in the internal capsule funnel down into the cerebral peduncle *(3).* The internal capsule also has a concave lateral surface; in this case the lenticular nucleus occupies the depression (see Figure 4-3, *F*).

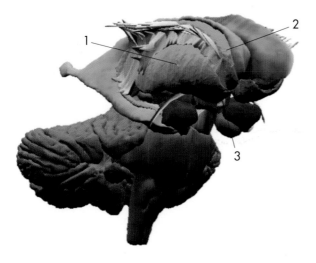

F, The lenticular nucleus *(1),* itself a combination of the putamen and the globus pallidus, occupies the depression in the internal capsule (see Figure 4-3, *E*). The putamen (the more lateral of the two) and the caudate nucleus *(2)* are actually continuous masses of gray matter. The area of continuity is called the nucleus accumbens *(3).* The amygdala *(red)* is a collection of nuclei underlying the medial surface of the temporal lobe at the anterior end of the hippocampus.

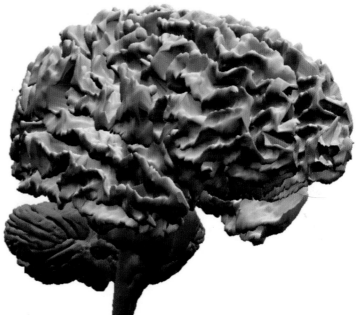

G, The structures described thus far are enveloped in white matter, containing the many millions of axons interconnecting different cortical areas or interconnecting the cortex and subcortical structures. This reconstruction shows the junction between the cerebral cortex and its underlying white matter.

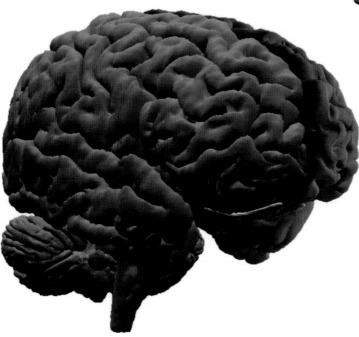

H, Finally, a thin (1.5 to 4.5 mm) layer of cerebral cortex covers each hemisphere.

chapter 5

CORONAL SECTIONS

This is the first of three chapters showing sections of entire human brains, in this case illustrating approximately coronal planes. Forebrain structures are emphasized, but parts of the brainstem and cerebellum are indicated as well. The organization of various functional systems in the forebrain (e.g., thalamus, hippocampus) is presented in Chapter 8.

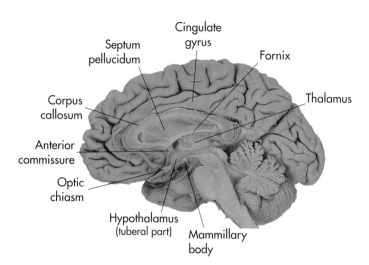

FIGURE 5-1
The hemisected brain from Figure 1-6, used in much of this chapter to indicate planes of section.

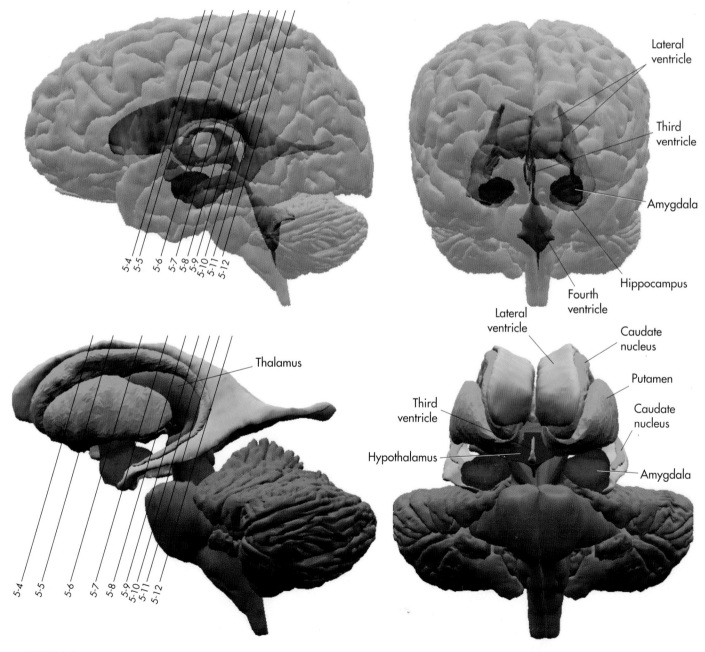

FIGURE 5-2
The planes of section shown in this chapter, indicated on three-dimensional reconstructions. (*Courtesy of Dr. John W. Sundsten, Department of Biological Structure, University of Washington School of Medicine*).

FIGURE 5-3
Twenty-four coronal sections of a brain, arranged in an anterior-to-posterior sequence from the anterior edge of the corpus callosum to the middle of the occipital lobe.

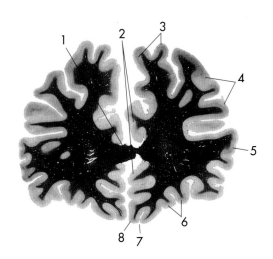

A, Anterior end of the genu of the corpus callosum *(1).* Convolutions that comprise most of the frontal lobe are the superior *(3),* middle *(4),* and inferior *(5)* frontal gyri, orbital gyri *(6),* and gyrus rectus *(8).* The cingulate gyrus *(2)* is cut twice, once above and once below the genu of the corpus callosum. The olfactory sulcus *(7),* which will be occupied by the olfactory tract at a slightly more posterior level, lies just lateral to the gyrus rectus.

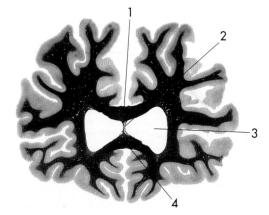

B, The anterior horn of the lateral ventricle *(3)* appears. A septum pellucidum *(2)* forms the medial wall of each lateral ventricle. The corpus callosum is now cut in two places, once through its body *(1)* above the septum pellucidum and once through its rostrum *(4)* below the septum pellucidum.

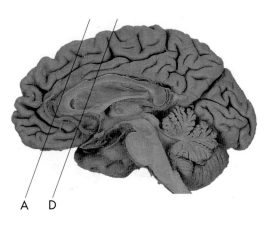

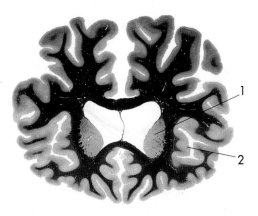

C, The head of the caudate nucleus *(1)* appears in the lateral wall of the lateral ventricle. The anterior region of the insula *(2)* is also visible at this level, overlying the caudate nucleus.

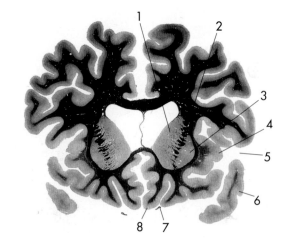

D, The rostral end of the putamen *(3)* is separated from the head of the caudate nucleus *(1)* by the anterior limb of the internal capsule *(2).* The putamen, the larger of the two parts of the lenticular nucleus, is overlain for its entire extent by the insula *(4).* The olfactory tract *(7)* lies in the olfactory sulcus, just lateral to gyrus rectus *(8).* The section passes through the tip of the temporal lobe *(6),* separated from the frontal lobe by the lateral sulcus *(5).*

FIGURE 5-3, cont'd.
Coronal sections.

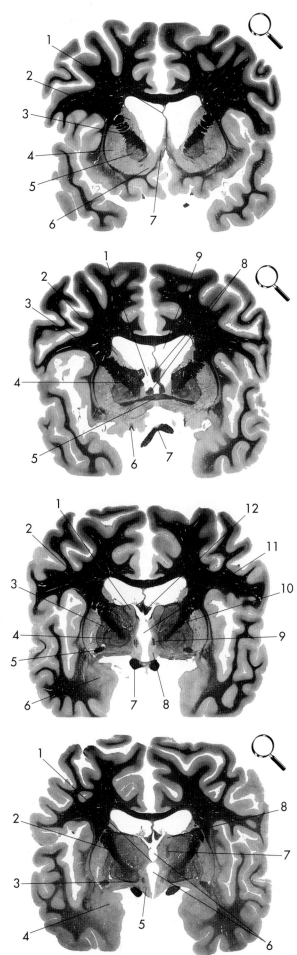

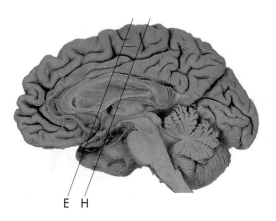

E, The globus pallidus (5) makes its appearance medial to the putamen (4); the two together comprise the lenticular nucleus. Nucleus accumbens (6), the region of continuity between the putamen and the head of the caudate nucleus, is also apparent. The septum pellucidum (1) is continuous with the septal nuclei (7). (The proximity of the nucleus accumbens to the septal nuclei was reflected in its earlier but now outmoded name—nucleus accumbens septi— "the nucleus leaning against the septum.") The anterior limb of the internal capsule (3) still occupies the cleft between the lenticular nucleus and the head of the caudate nucleus (2). Shown enlarged in Figure 5-4.

F, The level of the interventricular foramen (1) and anterior commissure (5) is a transition point for many structures, for example, from the head to the body of the caudate nucleus (2) and from the anterior horn to the body of the lateral ventricle (9). This section shaves off the anterior end of the thalamus (3), passes through the genu of the internal capsule (4), and cuts the fornix twice (8) as it curves ventrally toward the hypothalamus. The olfactory tract (6) joins the base of the forebrain, and the optic chiasm (7) appears. Shown enlarged in Figure 5-5.

G, Anterior diencephalon. Characteristic diencephalic features include the third ventricle (11), hypothalamus (8), and thalamic nuclei—anterior (1) and ventral anterior (2). The external (3) and internal (4) segments of the globus pallidus are now apparent, as is the anterior end of the amygdala (6). Fibers that will cross in the anterior commissure (5) accumulate beneath the lenticular nucleus. The fornix is cut twice, through the body (12) and column (9). The optic tract (7) and posterior limb of the internal capsule (10) are also present.

H, The mammillothalamic tract (7) enters the anterior nucleus (8) of the thalamus. The two thalami fuse at the interthalamic adhesion (1) or massa intermedia, which bridges the third ventricle (6). The ansa lenticularis (3, literally the "handle of the lenticular nucleus") emerges from the inferior surface of the globus pallidus and hooks around the posterior limb of the internal capsule (2). The amygdala (4) is larger and the middle of the three zones of the hypothalamus (the tuberal zone, 5) is present. Shown enlarged in Figure 5-6.

FIGURE 5-3, cont'd.
Coronal sections.

I, Additional efferents from the globus pallidus penetrate the posterior limb of the internal capsule *(2)* as the lenticular fasciculus and collect on the other side *(1)* before entering the thalamus. The column of the fornix *(4)* continues through the hypothalamus, where it will soon end in the mammillary body. The surface of the temporal lobe includes the superior *(3)*, middle *(5)*, and inferior *(6)* temporal gyri, and the occipitotemporal *(7)* and parahippocampal *(8)* gyri. The amygdala *(9)* has reached nearly maximal size.

J, Midthalamus. The dorsomedial *(2)* and ventrolateral *(3)* nuclei are prominent at this level. The optic tract *(6)* proceeds posteriorly toward its thalamic termination in the lateral geniculate nucleus. The column of the fornix is ending in the mammillary body *(10)*, which in turn gives rise to the mammillothalamic tract *(9)*. The lateral ventricle is another in a series of forebrain structures to be cut twice, here through the body *(1)* and through the inferior horn *(8)*, which has appeared adjacent to the amygdala *(7)*. Both the putamen *(4)* and the globus pallidus *(5)* begin to get smaller.

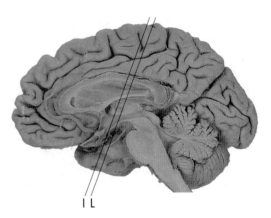

K, Level of the mammillary bodies *(6)*. Efferents from the globus pallidus and cerebellum collect beneath the thalamus in the thalamic fasciculus *(2)* before moving dorsally into the ventral lateral *(1)* and ventral anterior (see Figure 5-3, *G*) nuclei. The appropriately named subthalamic nucleus *(3)* appears beneath the thalamus. The amygdala *(4)* begins to get smaller and the hippocampus *(5)* assumes a position adjacent to the inferior horn of the lateral ventricle. Shown enlarged in Figure 5-7.

L, Brainstem structures begin to appear. The rostral end of the substantia nigra *(8)* is adjacent to the subthalamic nucleus *(9)*. Many fibers in the posterior limb of the internal capsule *(3)* continue into the cerebral peduncle *(7)*. Several structures are now cut twice, such as the body *(1)* and inferior horn *(6)* of the lateral ventricle and the body *(2)* and tail *(4)* of the caudate nucleus. The hippocampus *(5)* has almost completely replaced the amygdala on the right side of the section; the fornix *(10)*, the principal output bundle of the hippocampus, proceeds anteriorly in its characteristic trajectory medial to the lateral ventricle.

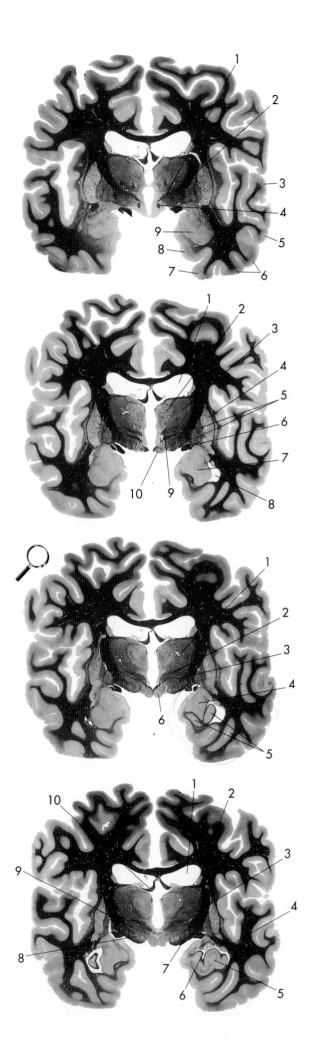

FIGURE 5-3, cont'd.
Coronal sections.

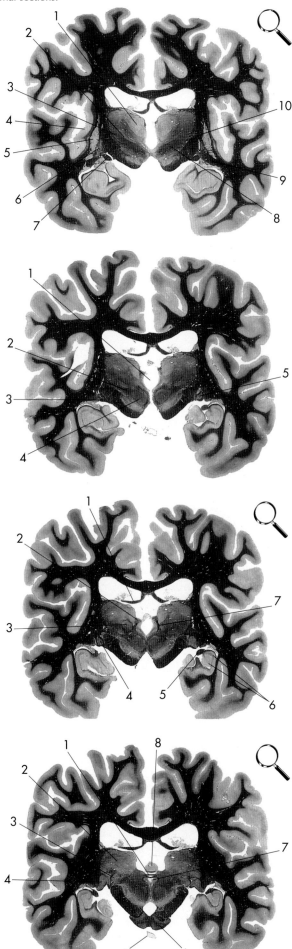

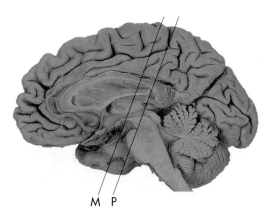

M, The dorsomedial *(1),* ventral posteromedial *(2),* and ventral posterolateral *(3)* nuclei now account for most of the thalamus. The putamen *(5)* and globus pallidus *(6)* continue to get smaller, as does the overlying insula *(4).* Cerebellar efferents *(8)* proceed rostrally toward the ventral lateral nucleus of the thalamus (see Figure 5-3, *K*), and the optic tract *(7)* continues posteriorly toward the lateral geniculate nucleus. The posterior limb *(10)* and sublenticular part *(9)* of the internal capsule partially surround the lenticular nucleus. Shown enlarged in Figure 5-8.

N, Posterior to the lenticular nucleus, the third ventricle *(1)* is smaller as the plane of section gets closer to the cerebral aqueduct. Cerebellar efferents *(2)* that have passed through or around the red nucleus *(4)* collect beneath the thalamus. The optic tract *(3)* begins to terminate in the lateral geniculate nucleus *(5)* on the right side of the section.

O, Near the diencephalon–midbrain junction, the lateral geniculate nucleus *(4)* is present on both sides, and the largest of the thalamic intralaminar nuclei, the centromedian nucleus *(3),* is apparent. The habenula *(2)* gives rise to the habenulointerpeduncular tract *(7).* Fornix fibers are again cut twice, this time where they are suspended from the corpus callosum as the posterior part of the body *(1)* and where they are still attached to the hippocampus *(6)* as the fimbria *(5).* Shown enlarged in Figure 5-9.

P, Posterior commissure *(1),* at the diencephalon–midbrain junction. The third ventricle has been replaced by the cerebral aqueduct *(7)* and a bit of the basal pons *(6)* appears, accompanied by the basilar artery *(5).* The only parts of the thalamus left are the pulvinar *(2)* and the medial *(3)* and lateral *(4)* geniculate nuclei. The pineal gland *(8)* is in the midline just above the posterior commissure. Shown enlarged in Figure 5-10.

FIGURE 5-3, cont'd.
Coronal sections.

Q, Posterior thalamus. Only the pulvinar *(6)* and the medial geniculate nucleus *(9)* remain. The plane of section approaches the posterior edge of C-shaped telencephalic structures, so the two parts of twice-cut structures draw closer together—the crus *(13)* and fimbria *(12)*, the body *(5)* and tail *(7)* of the caudate nucleus, the body *(4)* and inferior horn *(8)* of the lateral ventricle. Several brainstem structures are apparent, including the aqueduct *(2)* surrounded by periaqueductal gray *(3)*, the medial lemniscus *(10)* and the superior cerebellar peduncle *(11)*. The pineal gland *(1)* is still present above the most rostral part of the midbrain (the pretectal area). Shown enlarged in Figure 5-11.

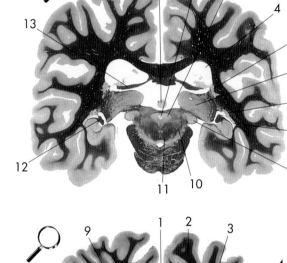

R, Splenium of the corpus callosum *(1)*. The section passes tangentially through the posterior edge of the caudate nucleus *(8)*, through fibers of the fornix as they pass from the fimbria *(5)* into the crus *(3)*, and through the lateral ventricle as the body *(4)* joins the inferior horn *(6)*. The superior colliculus *(9)* and the decussation of the superior cerebellar peduncles *(7)* can be seen in the brainstem. A little piece of the pulvinar *(2)* is all that remains of the thalamus. Shown enlarged in Figure 5-12.

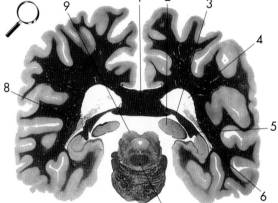

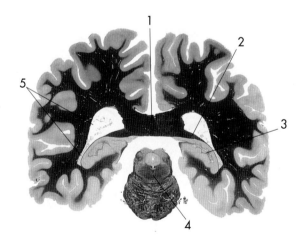

S, Now the section passes tangentially through the posterior end of the hippocampus *(3)* as it curves up underneath the splenium of the corpus callosum *(1)* and through the crus *(2)* of the fornix, the atrium *(5)* of the lateral ventricle, and the decussation of the superior cerebellar peduncles *(4)*.

T, Posterior edge of the splenium of the corpus callosum *(1)*. The section passes through choroid plexus *(7)* projecting back into the posterior horn of the lateral ventricle, and through remnants of the hippocampus *(2)*. The cerebellar hemispheres *(4)* begin to appear, the lateral lemniscus *(3)* ends in the inferior colliculus *(6)* and the trigeminal nerve *(5)* is attached to the pons.

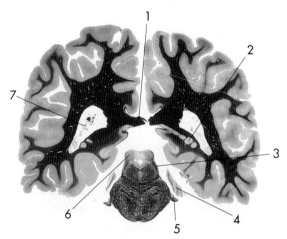

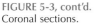

FIGURE 5-3, cont'd.
Coronal sections.

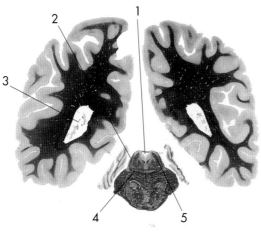

U, Choroid plexus *(3)* still protrudes into the posterior horn of the lateral ventricle. The aqueduct *(1)* begins to enlarge into the rostral part of the fourth ventricle. The lateral *(2)* and medial *(4)* lemnisci and the superior cerebellar peduncle *(5)* are apparent in the pons.

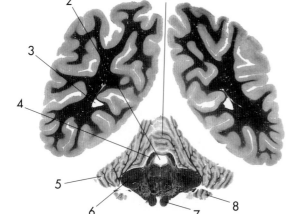

V, Last bit of the posterior horn of the lateral ventricle *(3)*. The cerebellar vermis *(1)*, hemispheres *(5)*, and flocculus *(8)* can now be distinguished. The aqueduct has opened into the fourth ventricle *(2)*, and the superior *(4)* and middle *(6)* cerebellar peduncles and the pyramid *(7)* are present.

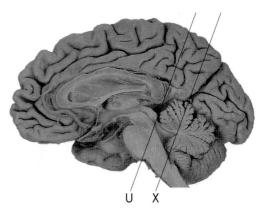

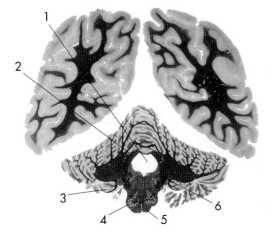

W, Pons and medulla. The fourth ventricle *(1)* is large, the pyramid *(5)* is massive, and the inferior olivary nucleus *(4)* is now present. The superior cerebellar peduncle *(2)* leaves the cerebellum and the inferior cerebellar peduncle *(6)* enters. The cerebellar flocculus *(3)* is still located adjacent to the pontomedullary junction.

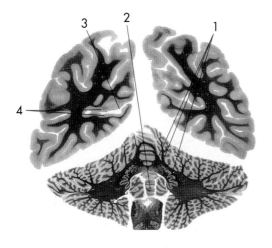

X, Deep cerebellar nuclei *(1)* and nodulus *(2)*. The calcarine sulcus *(3)*, with visual cortex in its upper and lower banks *(4)*, deeply indents the medial surface of the occipital lobe. (Note: the lower edge of the medulla was inadvertently detached during processing, so the pyramids are missing.)

FIGURE 5-4
A, A coronal section at the level of the anterior limb of the internal capsule. Actual size.

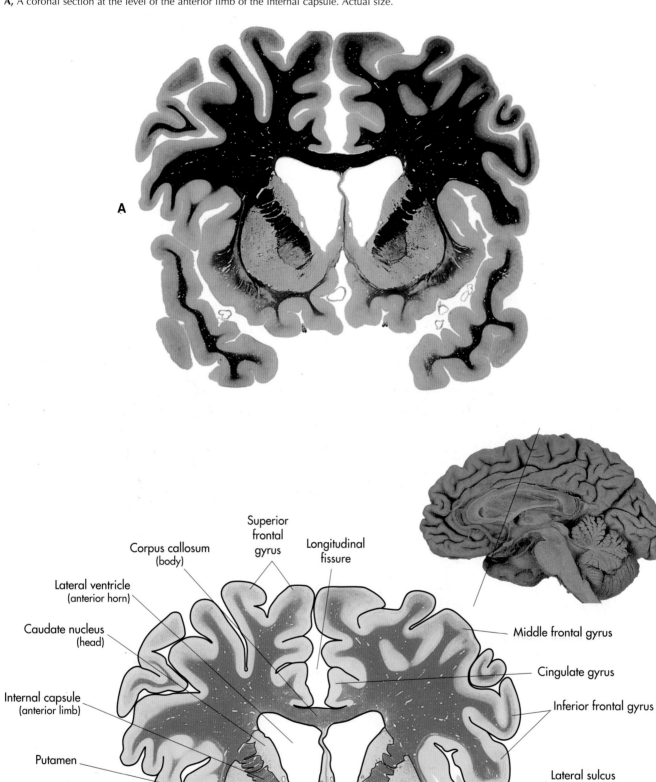

Superior frontal gyrus

Corpus callosum (body)

Longitudinal fissure

Lateral ventricle (anterior horn)

Caudate nucleus (head)

Internal capsule (anterior limb)

Putamen

Insula

Globus pallidus

Middle cerebral artery

Olfactory tract

Anterior cerebral artery

Middle frontal gyrus

Cingulate gyrus

Inferior frontal gyrus

Lateral sulcus

Superior temporal gyrus

Middle temporal gyrus

Inferior temporal gyrus

FIGURE 5-4, cont'd.
B, The central region of Figure 5-4, *A,* enlarged 1.5×.

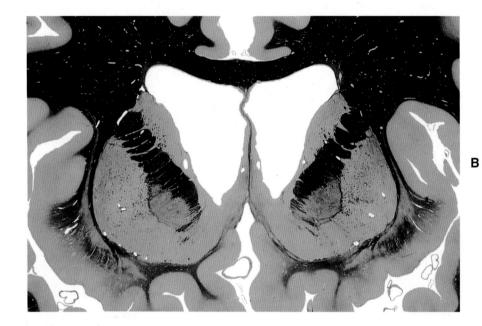

B

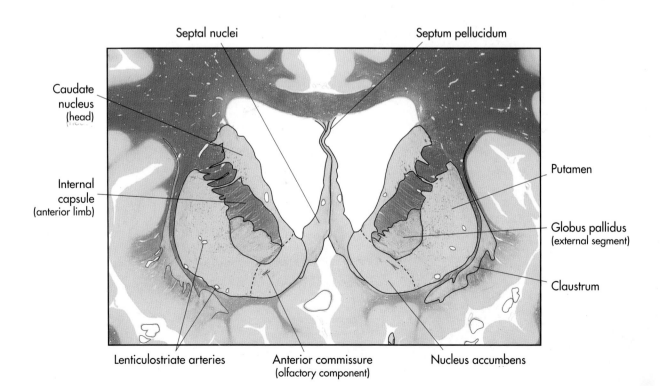

Septal nuclei

Septum pellucidum

Caudate
nucleus
(head)

Internal
capsule
(anterior limb)

Putamen

Globus pallidus
(external segment)

Claustrum

Lenticulostriate arteries

Anterior commissure
(olfactory component)

Nucleus accumbens

FIGURE 5-5
A, A coronal section at the level of the anterior commissure. Actual size.

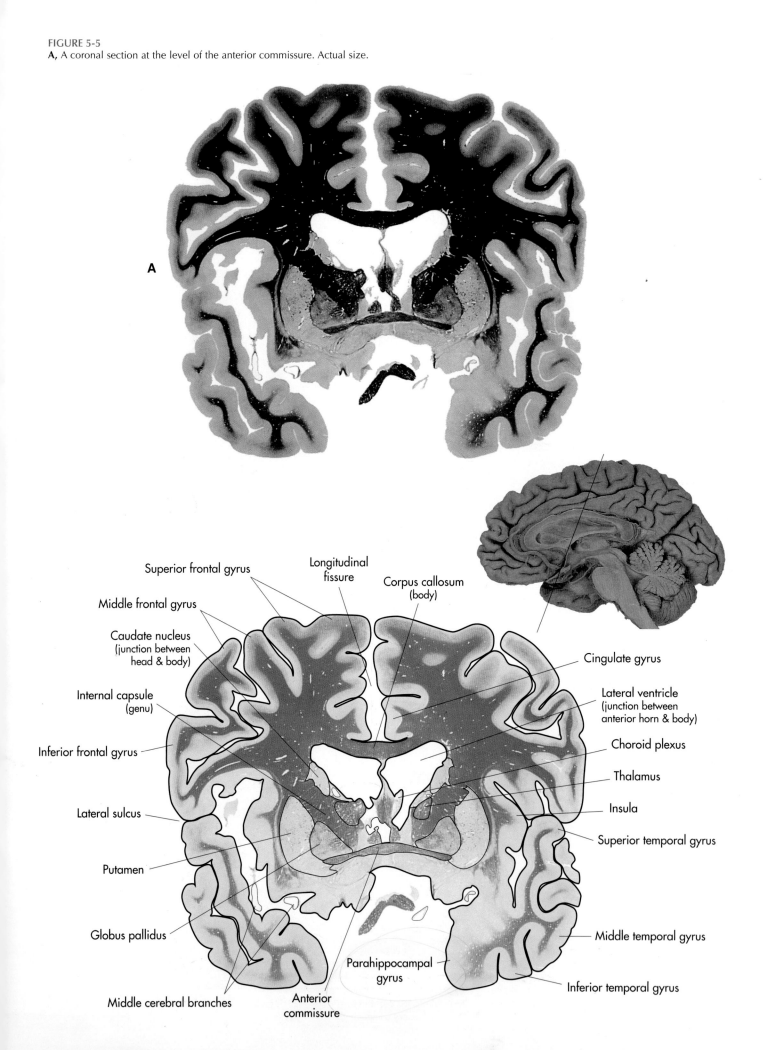

A

Superior frontal gyrus

Middle frontal gyrus

Caudate nucleus
(junction between
head & body)

Internal capsule
(genu)

Inferior frontal gyrus

Lateral sulcus

Putamen

Globus pallidus

Middle cerebral branches

Longitudinal
fissure

Corpus callosum
(body)

Cingulate gyrus

Lateral ventricle
(junction between
anterior horn & body)

Choroid plexus

Thalamus

Insula

Superior temporal gyrus

Middle temporal gyrus

Inferior temporal gyrus

Parahippocampal
gyrus

Anterior
commissure

FIGURE 5-5, cont'd.
B, The central region of Figure 5-5, *A,* enlarged 1.5×.

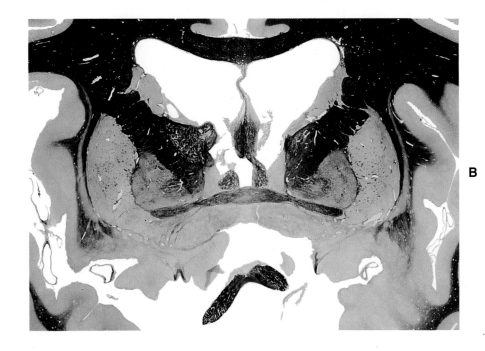

B

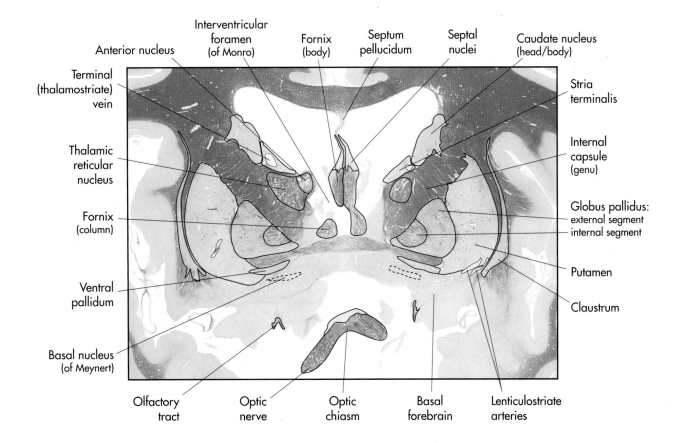

Anterior nucleus

Interventricular foramen (of Monro)

Fornix (body)

Septum pellucidum

Septal nuclei

Caudate nucleus (head/body)

Terminal (thalamostriate) vein

Stria terminalis

Thalamic reticular nucleus

Internal capsule (genu)

Fornix (column)

Globus pallidus: external segment internal segment

Ventral pallidum

Putamen

Claustrum

Basal nucleus (of Meynert)

Olfactory tract

Optic nerve

Optic chiasm

Basal forebrain

Lenticulostriate arteries

FIGURE 5-6
A, A coronal section at the level of the ansa lenticularis and the anterior thalamus. Actual size.

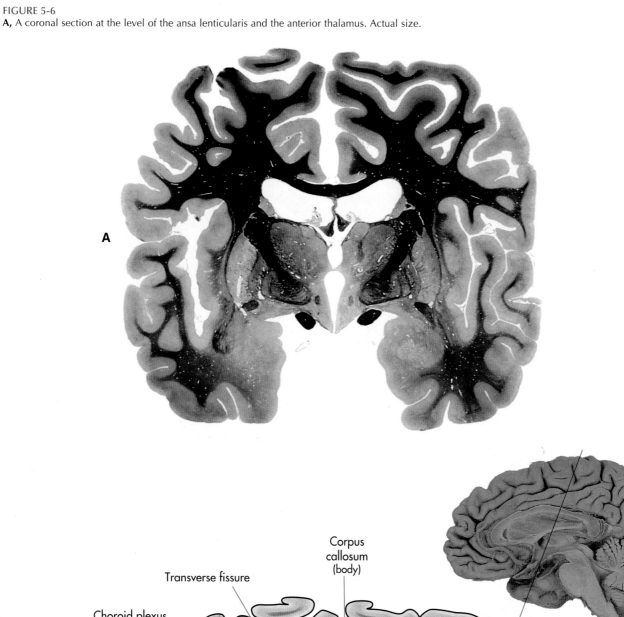

A

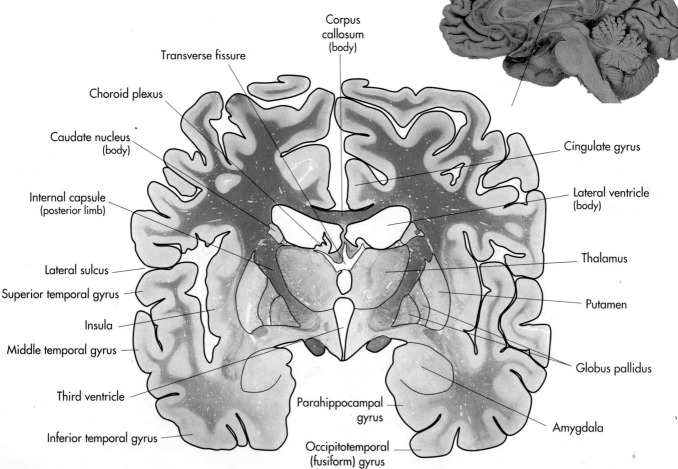

Corpus
callosum
(body)

Transverse fissure

Choroid plexus

Caudate nucleus
(body)

Cingulate gyrus

Internal capsule
(posterior limb)

Lateral ventricle
(body)

Lateral sulcus

Thalamus

Superior temporal gyrus

Putamen

Insula

Middle temporal gyrus

Globus pallidus

Third ventricle

Parahippocampal
gyrus

Amygdala

Inferior temporal gyrus

Occipitotemporal
(fusiform) gyrus

FIGURE 5-6, cont'd.
B, The central region of Figure 5-6, *A,* enlarged 1.5×.

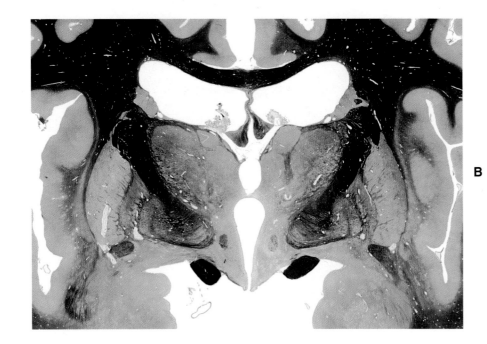

B

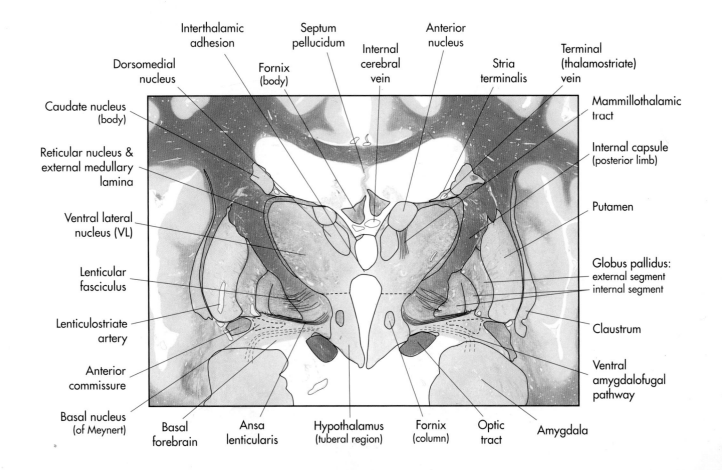

FIGURE 5-7
A, A coronal section at the level of the mammillary bodies. Actual size.

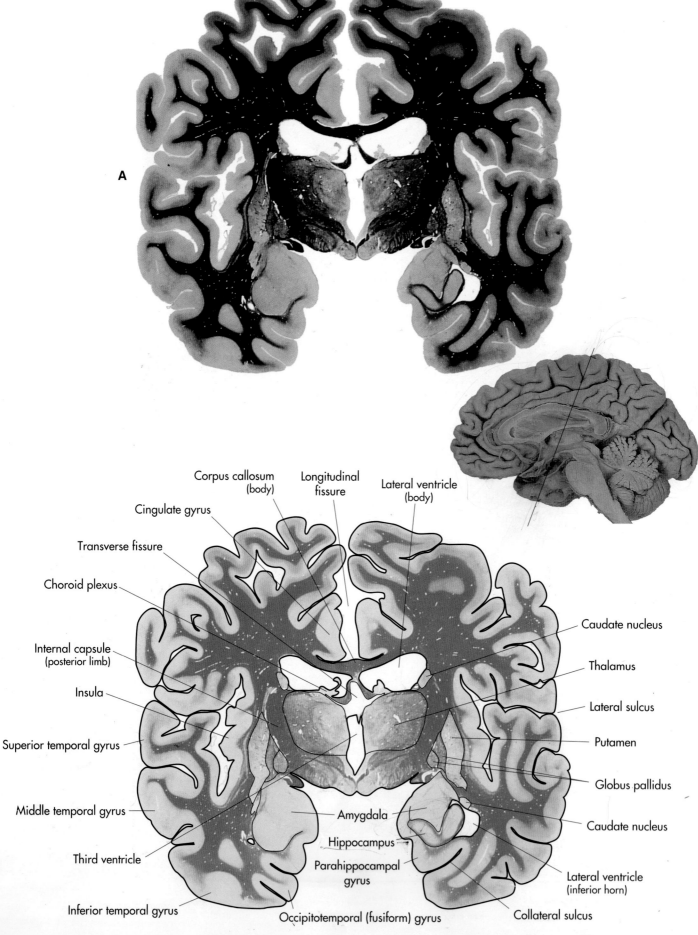

Corpus callosum (body)
Longitudinal fissure
Lateral ventricle (body)
Cingulate gyrus
Transverse fissure
Choroid plexus
Caudate nucleus
Internal capsule (posterior limb)
Thalamus
Insula
Lateral sulcus
Superior temporal gyrus
Putamen
Middle temporal gyrus
Globus pallidus
Amygdala
Caudate nucleus
Hippocampus
Third ventricle
Parahippocampal gyrus
Lateral ventricle (inferior horn)
Inferior temporal gyrus
Occipitotemporal (fusiform) gyrus
Collateral sulcus

FIGURE 5-7, cont'd.
B, The central region of Figure 5-7, *A,* enlarged 1.5×.

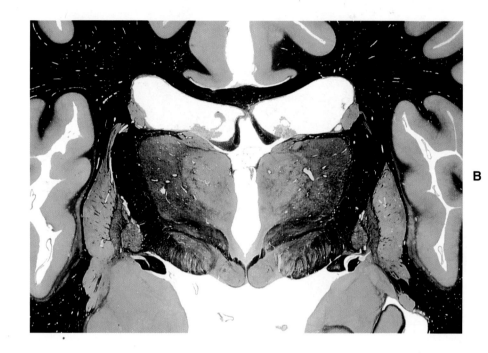

B

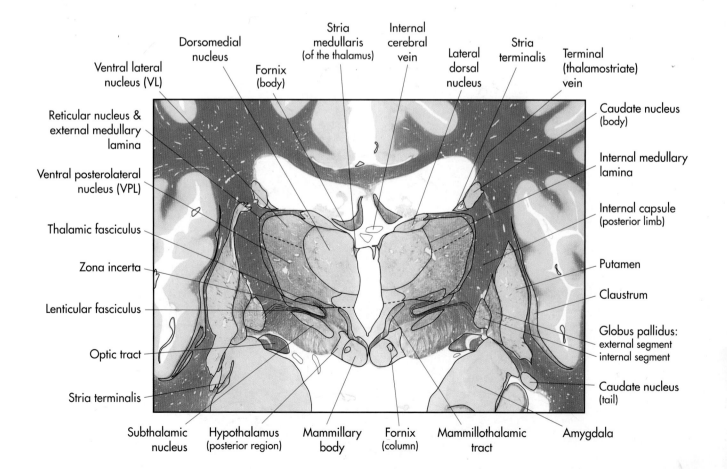

Ventral lateral nucleus (VL)

Dorsomedial nucleus

Fornix (body)

Stria medullaris (of the thalamus)

Internal cerebral vein

Lateral dorsal nucleus

Stria terminalis

Terminal (thalamostriate) vein

Reticular nucleus & external medullary lamina

Ventral posterolateral nucleus (VPL)

Thalamic fasciculus

Zona incerta

Lenticular fasciculus

Optic tract

Stria terminalis

Caudate nucleus (body)

Internal medullary lamina

Internal capsule (posterior limb)

Putamen

Claustrum

Globus pallidus: external segment internal segment

Caudate nucleus (tail)

Subthalamic nucleus

Hypothalamus (posterior region)

Mammillary body

Fornix (column)

Mammillothalamic tract

Amygdala

FIGURE 5-8
A, A coronal section at the level of the anterior end of the hippocampus. Actual size.

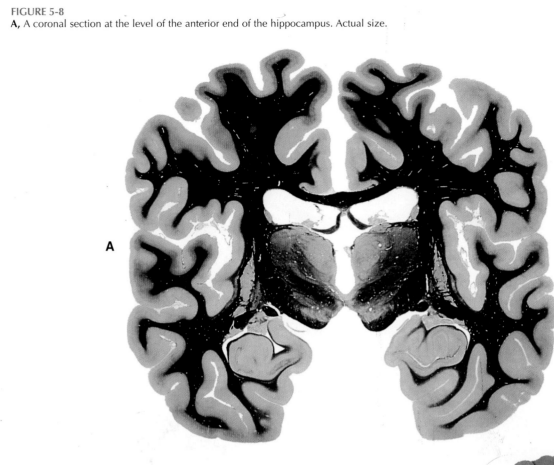

A

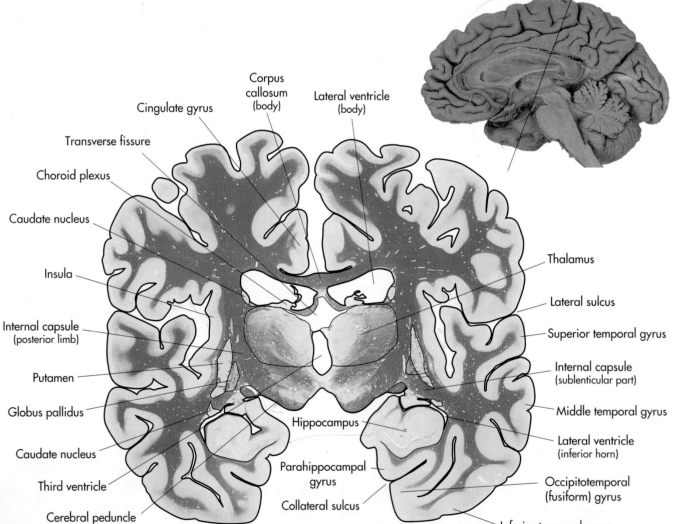

Cingulate gyrus

Corpus callosum (body)

Lateral ventricle (body)

Transverse fissure

Choroid plexus

Caudate nucleus

Insula

Internal capsule (posterior limb)

Putamen

Globus pallidus

Caudate nucleus

Third ventricle

Cerebral peduncle

Hippocampus

Parahippocampal gyrus

Collateral sulcus

Thalamus

Lateral sulcus

Superior temporal gyrus

Internal capsule (sublenticular part)

Middle temporal gyrus

Lateral ventricle (inferior horn)

Occipitotemporal (fusiform) gyrus

Inferior temporal gyrus

FIGURE 5-8, cont'd
B, The central region of Figure 5-8, *A,* enlarged 1.5×.

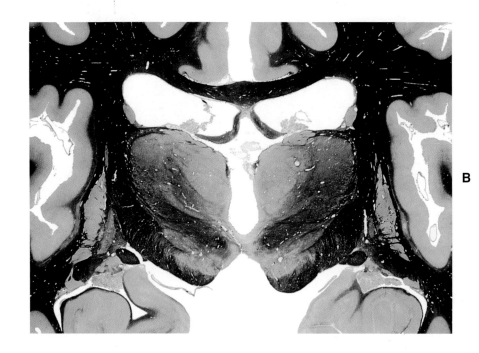

B

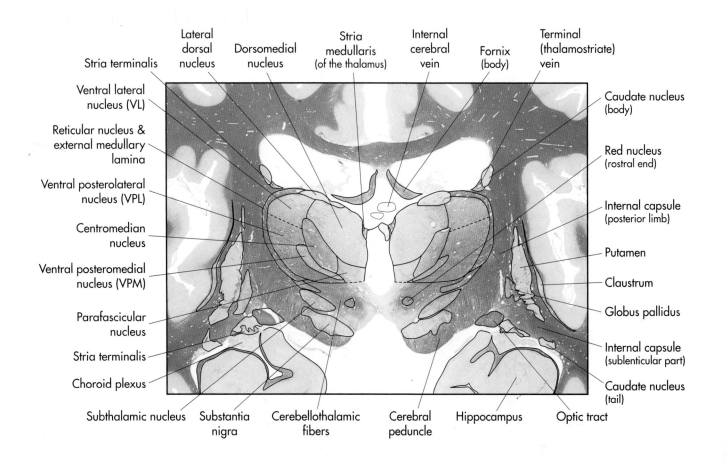

FIGURE 5-9
A, A coronal section through the posterior third of the thalamus. Actual size.

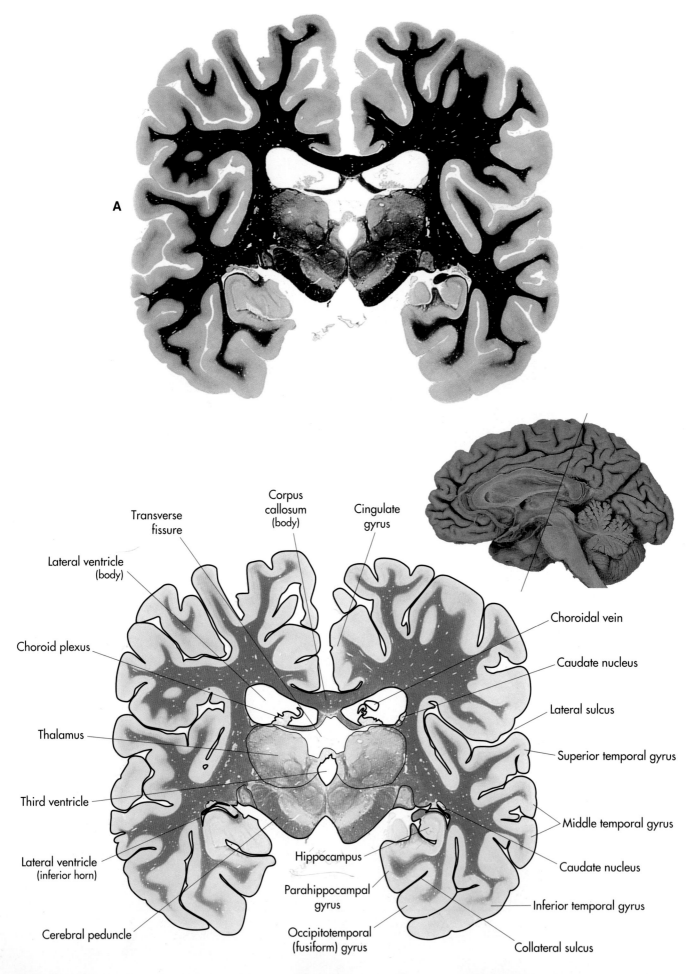

Transverse fissure

Corpus callosum (body)

Cingulate gyrus

Lateral ventricle (body)

Choroidal vein

Choroid plexus

Caudate nucleus

Lateral sulcus

Thalamus

Superior temporal gyrus

Third ventricle

Middle temporal gyrus

Lateral ventricle (inferior horn)

Hippocampus

Caudate nucleus

Parahippocampal gyrus

Inferior temporal gyrus

Cerebral peduncle

Occipitotemporal (fusiform) gyrus

Collateral sulcus

FIGURE 5-9, cont'd.
B, The central region of Figure 5-9, *A*, enlarged 1.5×.

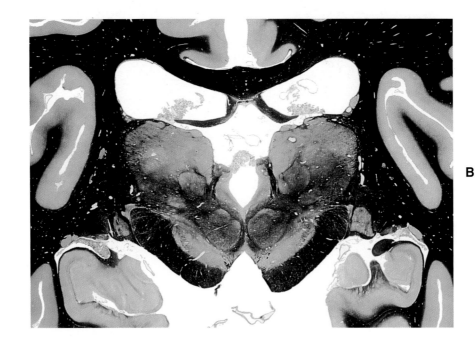

B

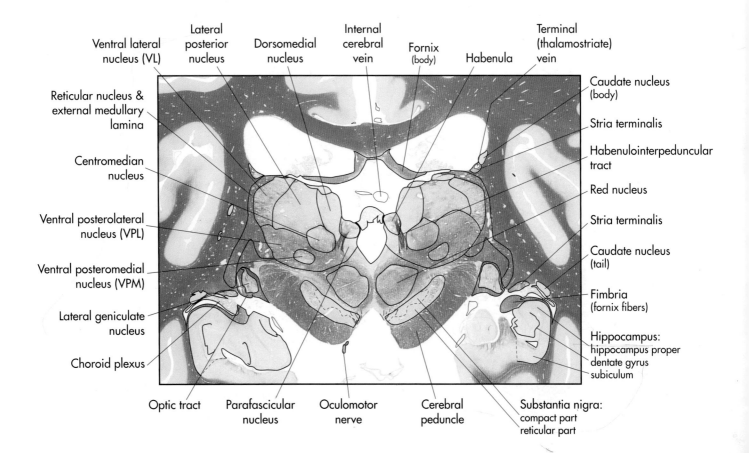

Ventral lateral nucleus (VL)

Lateral posterior nucleus

Dorsomedial nucleus

Internal cerebral vein

Fornix (body)

Habenula

Terminal (thalamostriate) vein

Reticular nucleus & external medullary lamina

Centromedian nucleus

Ventral posterolateral nucleus (VPL)

Ventral posteromedial nucleus (VPM)

Lateral geniculate nucleus

Choroid plexus

Caudate nucleus (body)

Stria terminalis

Habenulointerpeduncular tract

Red nucleus

Stria terminalis

Caudate nucleus (tail)

Fimbria (fornix fibers)

Hippocampus: hippocampus proper dentate gyrus subiculum

Optic tract

Parafascicular nucleus

Oculomotor nerve

Cerebral peduncle

Substantia nigra: compact part reticular part

FIGURE 5-10
A, A coronal section at the level of the posterior commissure. Actual size.

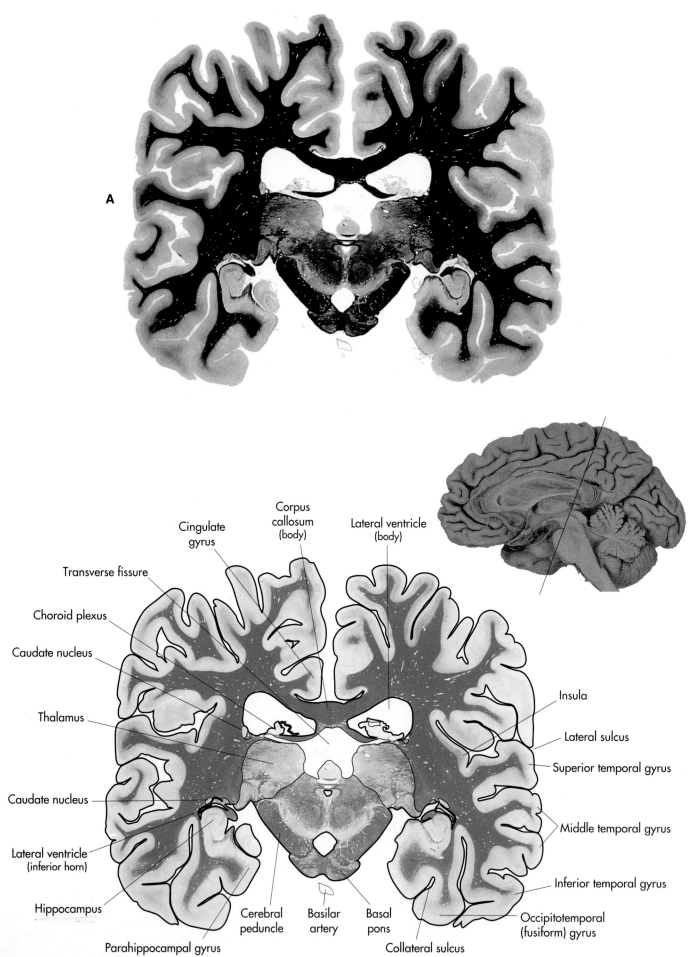

FIGURE 5-10, cont'd.
B, The central region of Figure 5-10, *A,* enlarged 1.5×.

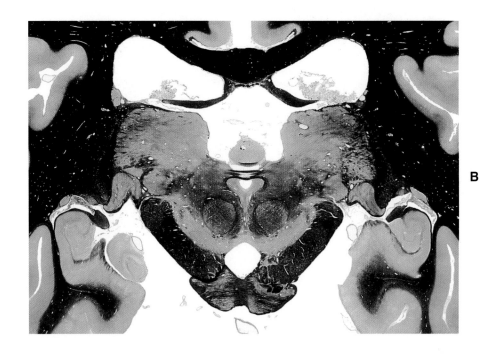

B

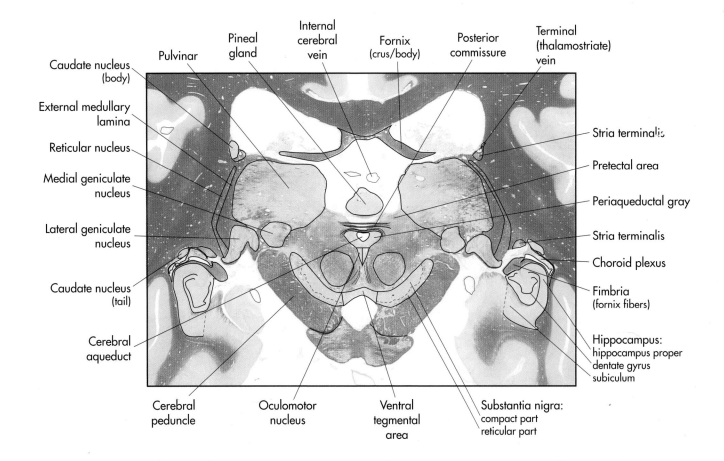

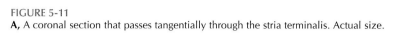

FIGURE 5-11
A, A coronal section that passes tangentially through the stria terminalis. Actual size.

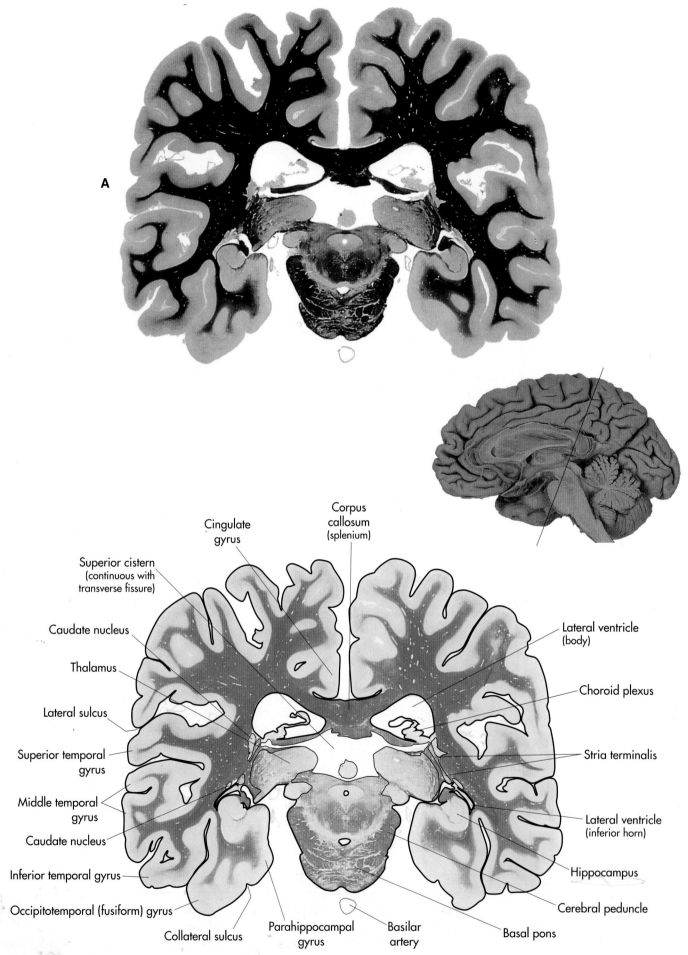

A

Cingulate gyrus

Corpus callosum (splenium)

Superior cistern (continuous with transverse fissure)

Caudate nucleus

Thalamus

Lateral sulcus

Superior temporal gyrus

Middle temporal gyrus

Caudate nucleus

Inferior temporal gyrus

Occipitotemporal (fusiform) gyrus

Collateral sulcus

Parahippocampal gyrus

Basilar artery

Lateral ventricle (body)

Choroid plexus

Stria terminalis

Lateral ventricle (inferior horn)

Hippocampus

Cerebral peduncle

Basal pons

FIGURE 5-11, cont'd.
B, The central region of Figure 5-11, *A,* enlarged 1.5×.

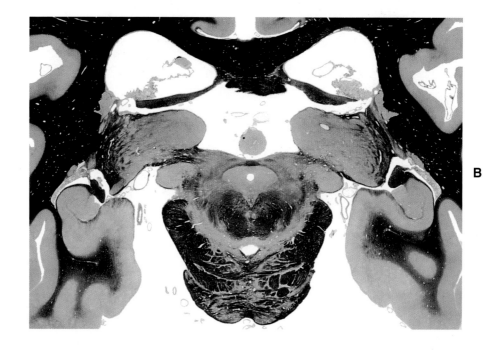

B

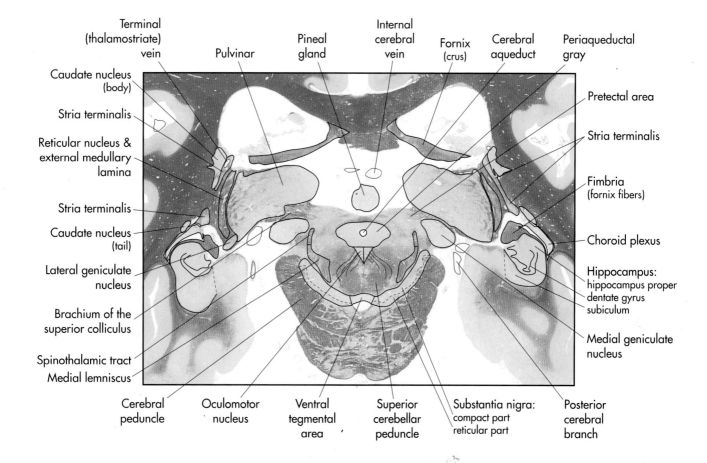

Terminal
(thalamostriate)
vein

Caudate nucleus
(body)

Stria terminalis

Reticular nucleus &
external medullary
lamina

Stria terminalis

Caudate nucleus
(tail)

Lateral geniculate
nucleus

Brachium of the
superior colliculus

Spinothalamic tract

Medial lemniscus

Pulvinar

Pineal
gland

Internal
cerebral
vein

Fornix
(crus)

Cerebral
aqueduct

Periaqueductal
gray

Pretectal area

Stria terminalis

Fimbria
(fornix fibers)

Choroid plexus

Hippocampus:
hippocampus proper
dentate gyrus
subiculum

Medial geniculate
nucleus

Cerebral
peduncle

Oculomotor
nucleus

Ventral
tegmental
area

Superior
cerebellar
peduncle

Substantia nigra:
compact part
reticular part

Posterior
cerebral
branch

FIGURE 5-12
A, A coronal section that passes tangentially through the fornix and caudate nucleus. Actual size.

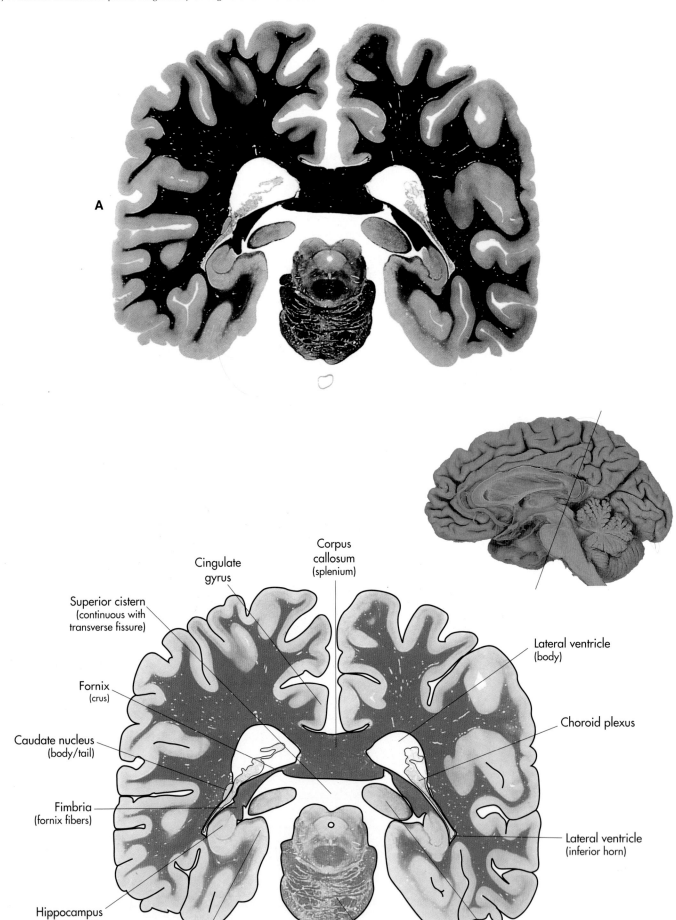

Cingulate
gyrus

Corpus
callosum
(splenium)

Superior cistern
(continuous with
transverse fissure)

Lateral ventricle
(body)

Fornix
(crus)

Caudate nucleus
(body/tail)

Choroid plexus

Fimbria
(fornix fibers)

Lateral ventricle
(inferior horn)

Hippocampus

Parahippocampal gyrus

Basilar
artery

Basal
pons

Thalamus

FIGURE 5-12, cont'd
B, The central region of Figure 5-12, *A,* enlarged 1.5×.

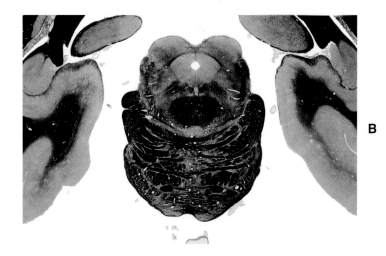

B

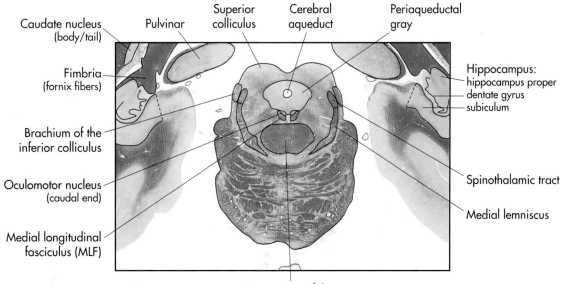

Caudate nucleus (body/tail)

Pulvinar

Superior colliculus

Cerebral aqueduct

Periaqueductal gray

Fimbria (fornix fibers)

Hippocampus: hippocampus proper dentate gyrus subiculum

Brachium of the inferior colliculus

Oculomotor nucleus (caudal end)

Spinothalamic tract

Medial lemniscus

Medial longitudinal fasciculus (MLF)

Decussation of the superior cerebellar peduncles

HORIZONTAL SECTIONS

This chapter, the second of three showing sections of entire human brains, illustrates approximately horizontal planes. Forebrain structures continue to be emphasized, but parts of the brainstem and cerebellum are indicated as well. The organization of various functional systems in the forebrain (e.g., thalamus, hippocampus) is presented in Chapter 8.

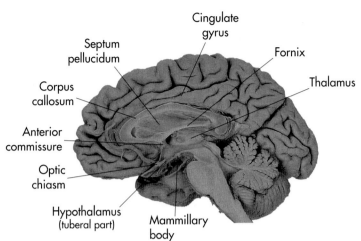

FIGURE 6-1
The hemisected brain from Figure 1-6, used in much of this chapter to indicate planes of section.

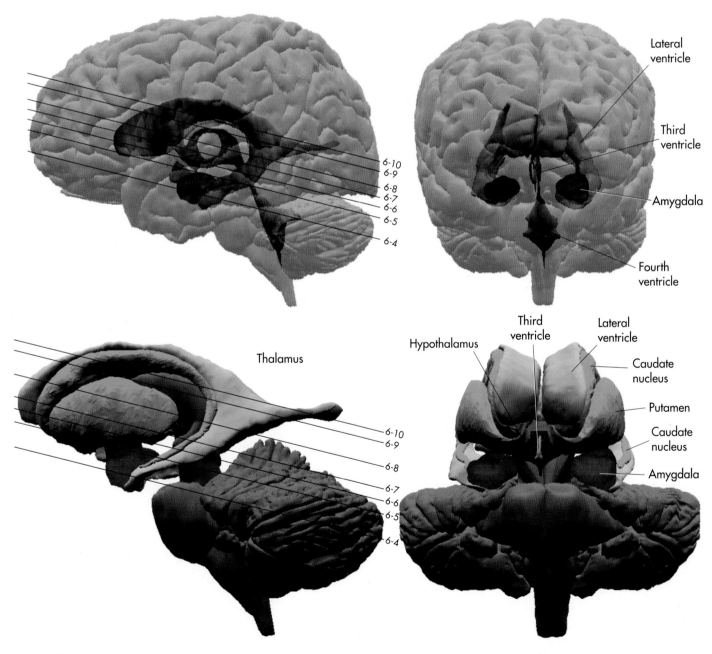

FIGURE 6-2
The planes of section shown in this chapter, indicated on three-dimensional reconstructions. *(Courtesy of Dr. John W. Sundsten, Department of Biological Structure, University of Washington School of Medicine.)*

67

FIGURE 6-3
Twenty-four horizontal sections of a brain, arranged in an inferior-to-superior sequence extending from the orbital surface of the frontal lobe to just above the corpus callosum. Anterior is toward the top, as in the conventional orientation of computed tomography (CT) and magnetic resonance (MR) images.

A, The first section just reaches the orbital surface of the frontal lobe, including gyrus rectus *(1),* and passes through the olfactory sulcus *(7)* and olfactory tract *(2).* The temporal pole *(3)* can also be seen. The brainstem is cut at an odd angle in these sections, with more rostral parts toward the top. This section passes through the basal pons *(4)* and the inferior olivary nucleus *(6)* of the medulla. The corticospinal tract *(5)* can be seen passing from the basal pons into the medullary pyramid.

B, Gyrus rectus *(1)* is still present and is now joined by a little more orbital frontal cortex. The section again passes through the basal pons *(3)* and the basilar artery *(2)* anterior to it, as well as parts of the rostral medulla. It includes the cerebellar flocculus *(4),* the inferior cerebellar peduncle *(5),* the trigeminal *(8)* and vestibulocochlear *(7)* nerves, and choroid plexus *(6)* in the lateral aperture of the fourth ventricle.

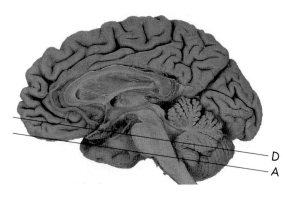

C, The olfactory tract *(1)* has now reached the posterior end of the olfactory sulcus, near where it attaches to the base of the forebrain. The optic nerve *(2)* moves posteriorly toward the optic chiasm; the internal carotid artery *(3)* is just lateral to where the optic chiasm will soon be located. The inferior horn of the lateral ventricle *(5)* and adjacent amygdala *(4)* begin to appear in the temporal lobe. The inferior cerebellar peduncle *(6)* turns posteriorly toward the cerebellum.

D, The middle cerebral artery *(1)* moves laterally into the lateral sulcus. The amygdala *(3)* is larger, and the hippocampus *(4)* appears; both structures underlie the uncus *(2).* The plane of section moves closer to the hypothalamus and passes through the infundibulum *(7).* The middle cerebellar peduncle *(5)* connects the basal pons to the cerebellum, and the abducens nerve *(6)* moves anteriorly from its point of emergence from the brainstem.

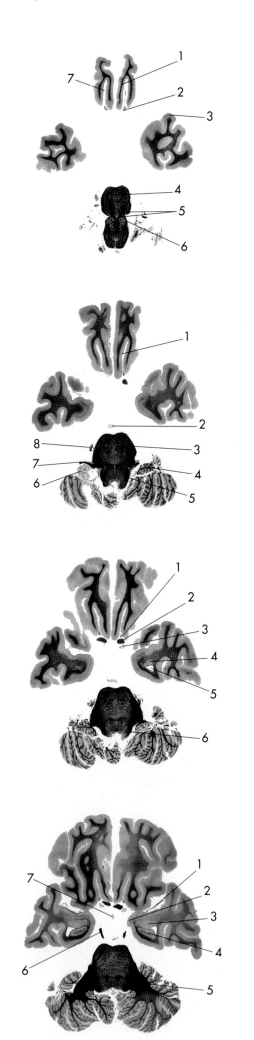

FIGURE 6-3, cont'd.
Horizontal sections.

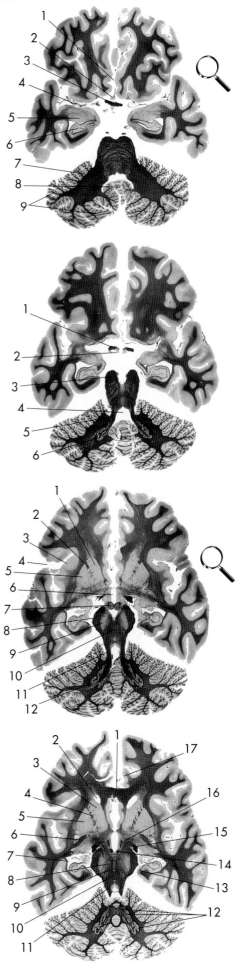

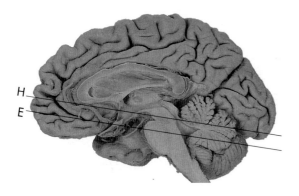

E, The anterior cerebral artery *(2)* moves into the longitudinal fissure *(1),* and the middle cerebral artery *(4)* continues on its course toward the insula. The optic nerves partially decussate in the optic chiasm *(3).* The amygdala *(5)* and hippocampus *(6)* continue to increase in size. The cerebellar vermis *(8)* and hemispheres *(9)* can be distinguished, and the middle cerebellar peduncle *(7)* still connects the basal pons to the cerebellum. Shown enlarged in Figure 6-4.

F, The optic tract *(1)* begins to move posteriorly from the optic chiasm, and the plane of section reaches the tuberal zone of the hypothalamus *(2).* The superior cerebellar peduncle *(5)* leaves the dentate nucleus *(6),* forms part of the wall of the fourth ventricle *(4),* and enters the pons. The first part of the midbrain to appear in this plane of section is the cerebral peduncle *(3).*

G, Base of the forebrain, beginning to pass through the head of the caudate nucleus *(1),* the putamen *(5),* and the anterior limb of the internal capsule *(2).* The insula *(3),* buried in the lateral sulcus *(4),* overlies the putamen. The mammillary bodies *(7)* and other parts of the hypothalamus border the third ventricle *(6).* The cerebral peduncle *(8)* and substantia nigra *(9)* are apparent in the midbrain. The superior cerebellar peduncle *(11)* leaves the dentate nucleus *(12),* enters the brainstem, and decussates *(10).* Shown enlarged in Figure 6-5.

H, The lateral ventricle is now cut twice, through the anterior *(2)* and inferior *(7)* horns, and the corpus callosum *(1)* makes its first appearance. The limbic lobe is also cut twice, through the cingulate *(17)* and parahippocampal *(13)* gyri. The head of the caudate nucleus *(3),* the putamen *(5),* and the anterior limb of the internal capsule *(4)* all increase in size. Fibers that will cross in the anterior commissure *(6)* begin to move toward the midline, and the optic tract *(15)* continues to move posteriorly. The column of the fornix *(16)* and the mammillothalamic tract *(14)* are transected just above each mammillary body. All of the deep cerebellar nuclei *(12)* are now apparent. The vast majority of efferents from these nuclei travel through the superior cerebellar peduncle *(11),* decussate *(10),* and then most of them *(9)* pass through or around the red nucleus *(8).*

FIGURE 6-3, cont'd.
Horizontal sections.

I, The subcallosal gyrus *(1)*, the last bit of limbic cortex adjacent to the corpus callosum, borders the longitudinal fissure *(12)*. The head of the caudate nucleus *(2)* continues; both parts of the lenticular nucleus—the putamen *(3)* and the globus pallidus *(4)*—are now apparent, and the subthalamic nucleus *(5)* can be seen just across the internal capsule from the globus pallidus. Fornix fibers are cut twice, once through the fimbria *(8)* as it leaves the hippocampus *(7)* and again through the column of the fornix *(10)* as it approaches the mammillary body. The mammillothalamic tract *(9)* continues on its course toward the anterior nucleus of the thalamus. Fibers of the anterior commissure *(11)* cross the midline. The dentate nucleus *(6)* is the only deep cerebellar nucleus remaining.

J, The section passes tangentially through the corpus callosum as the genu *(1)* merges with the rostrum *(2)*. The anterior commissure *(3)*, column of the fornix *(4)*, and subthalamic nucleus *(5)* are still visible, and the inferior colliculus *(6)* appears. Shown enlarged in Figure 6-6.

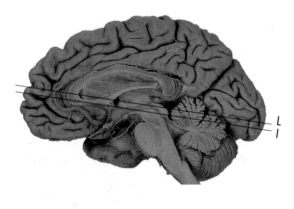

K, The septum pellucidum *(1)*, merging with the septal nuclei *(2)*, succeeds the rostrum of the corpus callosum. The lateral *(3)* and medial *(4)* geniculate nuclei (the most inferior parts of the thalamus) can now be seen, and the continuity of the third ventricle *(6)* and the cerebral aqueduct *(5)* is apparent.

L, Choroid plexus *(1)* passes through each interventricular foramen adjacent to the column of the fornix *(10)*. Four of the five parts of the internal capsule—the anterior limb *(2)*, genu *(3)*, posterior limb *(4)*, and retrolenticular part *(5)*—are now present, as is much more of the thalamus *(6)*. The mammillothalamic tract *(9)* continues on its path toward the anterior nucleus of the thalamus. The posterior commissure *(7)* crosses the midline near the periaqueductal gray *(8)*. Shown enlarged in Figure 6-7.

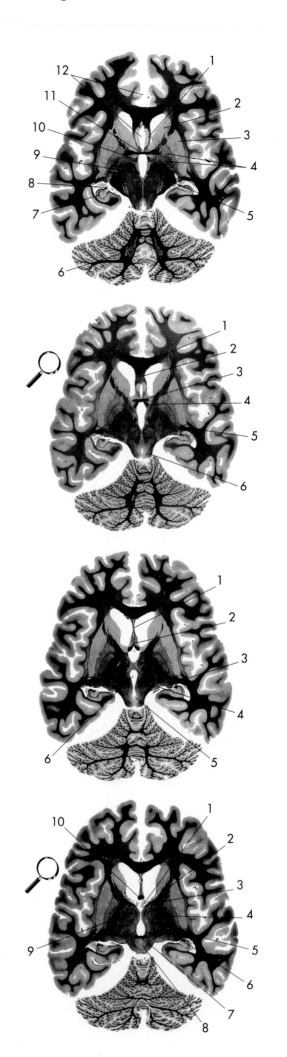

FIGURE 6-3, cont'd.
Horizontal sections.

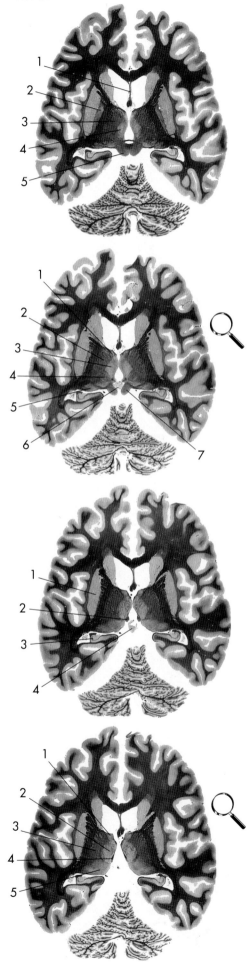

M, The septum pellucidum *(1)* still separates the anterior horns of the two lateral ventricles from each other. The globus pallidus *(2)* gets smaller as the plane of section moves superiorly through the lenticular nucleus. Lateral *(3)* and medial *(4)* divisions of the thalamus can be distinguished because of differences in the numbers of myelinated fibers entering and leaving them. The superior colliculus *(5)* appears in the midbrain.

N, Now more parts of the thalamus can be seen: the lateral *(2)* and medial *(3)* divisions, the anterior *(1)* and centromedian *(4)* nuclei, and the pulvinar *(5)*. (The mammillothalamic tract has terminated in the anterior nucleus and is no longer visible.) The pineal gland *(6)* protrudes posteriorly between the superior colliculi *(7)*. Shown enlarged in Figure 6-8.

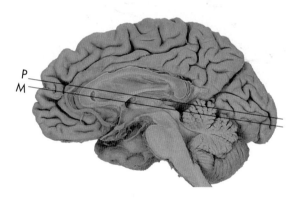

O, The plane of section is above the globus pallidus, and now the putamen *(1)* begins to get smaller. The stria medullaris of the thalamus terminates in the habenula *(2)*. The hippocampus *(3)* and pineal gland *(4)* are still apparent.

P, In the thalamus, lateral *(3)* and medial *(2)* divisions, the anterior nucleus *(1)*, and the pulvinar *(5)* can still be distinguished. Fibers travel posteriorly in the stria medullaris *(4)* of the thalamus toward the habenula. Shown enlarged in Figure 6-9.

FIGURE 6-3, cont'd.
Horizontal sections.

Q, The putamen *(3)* continues to get smaller, as does the overlying insula *(4).* As the plane of section moves upward through the cerebral hemisphere, the profiles of twice-cut structures, such as the lateral ventricle *(1, 6)* and fornix fibers *(2, 5),* will draw progressively closer to each other until these C-shaped structures are finally cut tangentially (e.g., *T, V*).

R, Near the top of the putamen *(3)* and internal capsule *(2).* The fornix *(1)* is now cut obliquely as it begins to curve downward toward the interventricular foramen. Although the thalamus *(4)* begins to get smaller, medial and lateral divisions, the anterior nucleus, and the pulvinar can still be distinguished.

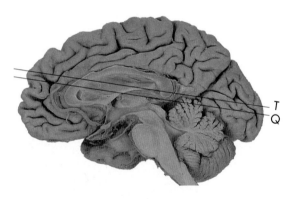

S, Just below the splenium of the corpus callosum and completely above the putamen. The head of the caudate nucleus *(1)* begins to taper into the body of the caudate nucleus, and the posterior part of the hippocampus *(5)* has a distinctive pattern of folding (compare to *R*). The plane of section still passes through the inferior horn *(4),* but will soon enter the atrium and posterior horn of the lateral ventricle. The fornix *(2)* is cut obliquely once again. The internal cerebral vein *(3)* travels posteriorly toward the great cerebral vein. Enlarged in Figure 6-10.

T, The corpus callosum is now cut twice, through the body *(9)* and the splenium *(4).* The thalamus *(3)* continues to dwindle, the distinctive appearance of the hippocampus *(7)* continues, and the two profiles of the lateral ventricle *(1, 6)* draw closer together. On the right side of the section, fornix fibers are still cut twice *(2, 5),* but on the left side the section cuts tangentially through these fibers *(8),* showing their entire course as they pass from the fimbria to the fornix.

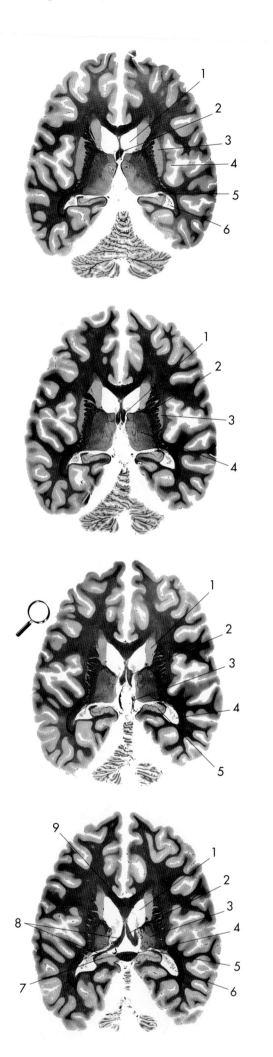

FIGURE 6-3, cont'd.
Horizontal sections.

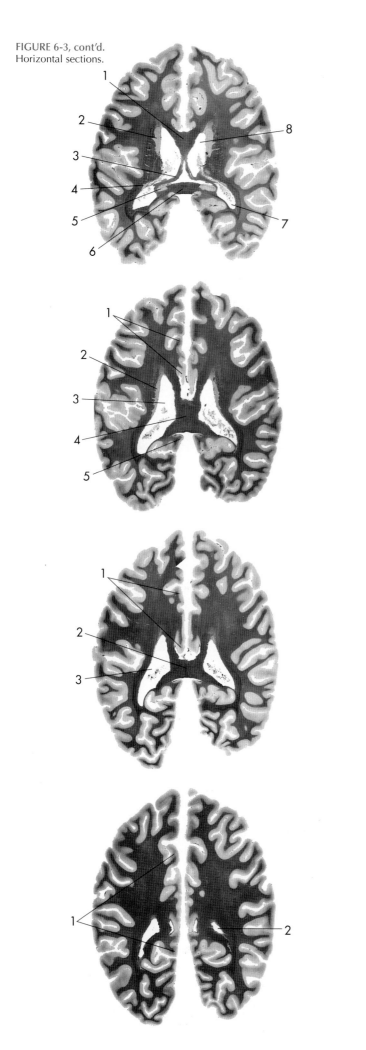

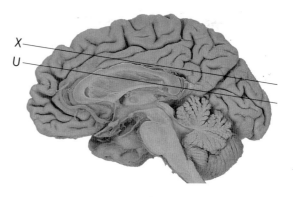

U, The plane of section has nearly reached the top of several C-shaped forebrain structures. It passes tangentially through the fornix *(3)*, but still cuts the corpus callosum *(1, 6)*, caudate nucleus *(2, 4)*, and lateral ventricle *(7, 8)* twice. The last bit of the hippocampus *(5)* can be seen adjacent to the splenium of the corpus callosum *(6)*.

V, A tangential section through the body of the caudate nucleus *(2)*, the lateral ventricle *(3)*, and the body of the corpus callosum *(4)*. The limbic lobe is still cut twice, once (nearly tangentially) through the cingulate gyrus *(1)* and again through the narrow isthmus *(5)* joining the cingulate and parahippocampal gyri.

W, A tangential cut through the corpus callosum *(2)*, lateral ventricle *(3)*, and a larger expanse of the cingulate gyrus *(1)*.

X, Finally, a tangential cut through the cingulate gyrus *(1)* just above the corpus callosum and near the roof of the lateral ventricle *(2)*.

FIGURE 6-4
A, A horizontal section through the uncus and optic chiasm. Three fourths actual size.

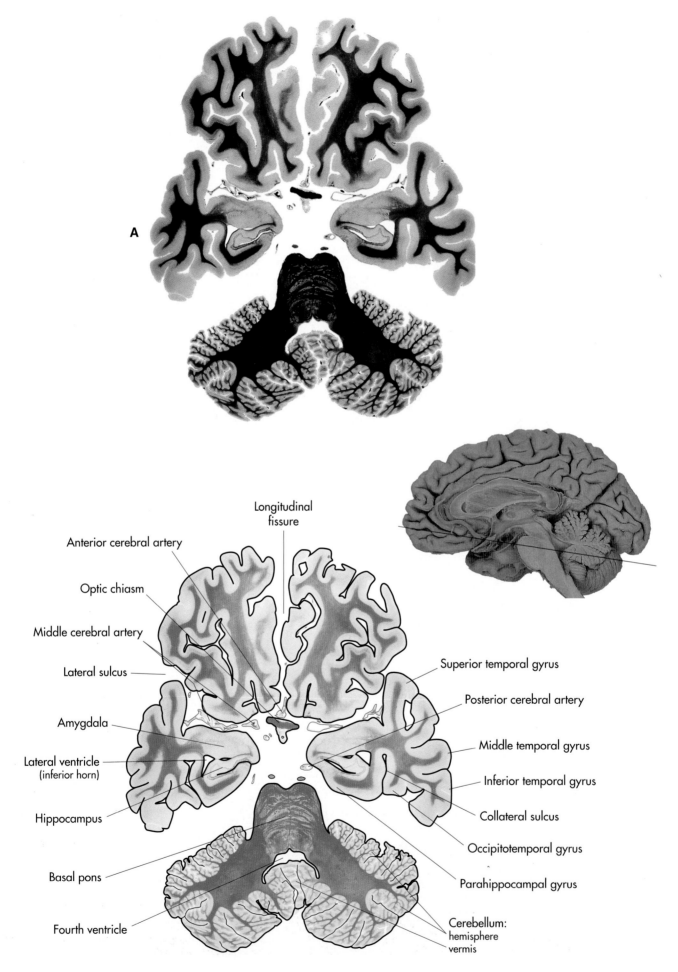

A

Longitudinal
fissure

Anterior cerebral artery

Optic chiasm

Middle cerebral artery

Lateral sulcus

Amygdala

Lateral ventricle
(inferior horn)

Hippocampus

Basal pons

Fourth ventricle

Superior temporal gyrus

Posterior cerebral artery

Middle temporal gyrus

Inferior temporal gyrus

Collateral sulcus

Occipitotemporal gyrus

Parahippocampal gyrus

Cerebellum:
hemisphere
vermis

FIGURE 6-4, cont'd.
B, The central region of Figure 6-4, *A,* enlarged to 1.5× actual size.

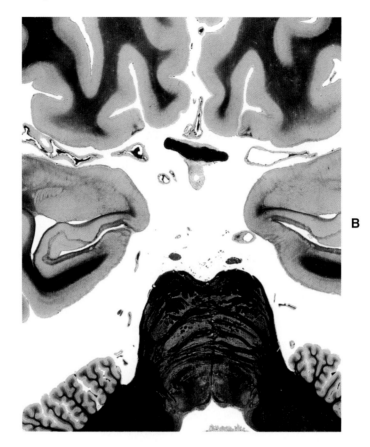

B

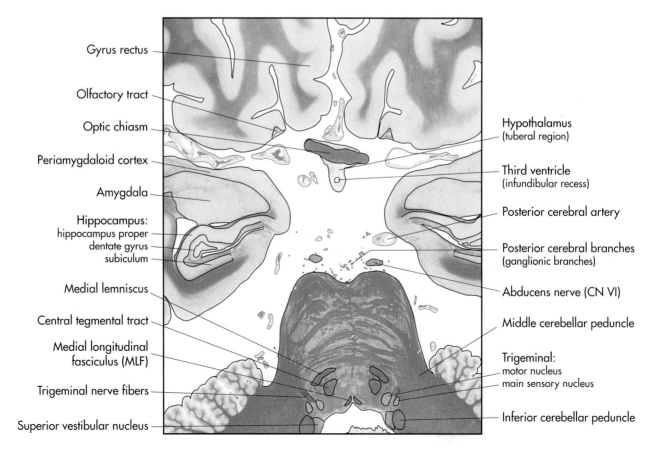

Gyrus rectus

Olfactory tract

Optic chiasm

Periamygdaloid cortex

Amygdala

Hippocampus:
hippocampus proper
dentate gyrus
subiculum

Medial lemniscus

Central tegmental tract

Medial longitudinal
fasciculus (MLF)

Trigeminal nerve fibers

Superior vestibular nucleus

Hypothalamus
(tuberal region)

Third ventricle
(infundibular recess)

Posterior cerebral artery

Posterior cerebral branches
(ganglionic branches)

Abducens nerve (CN VI)

Middle cerebellar peduncle

Trigeminal:
motor nucleus
main sensory nucleus

Inferior cerebellar peduncle

FIGURE 6-5
A, A horizontal section through the base of the diencephalon. Three fourths actual size.

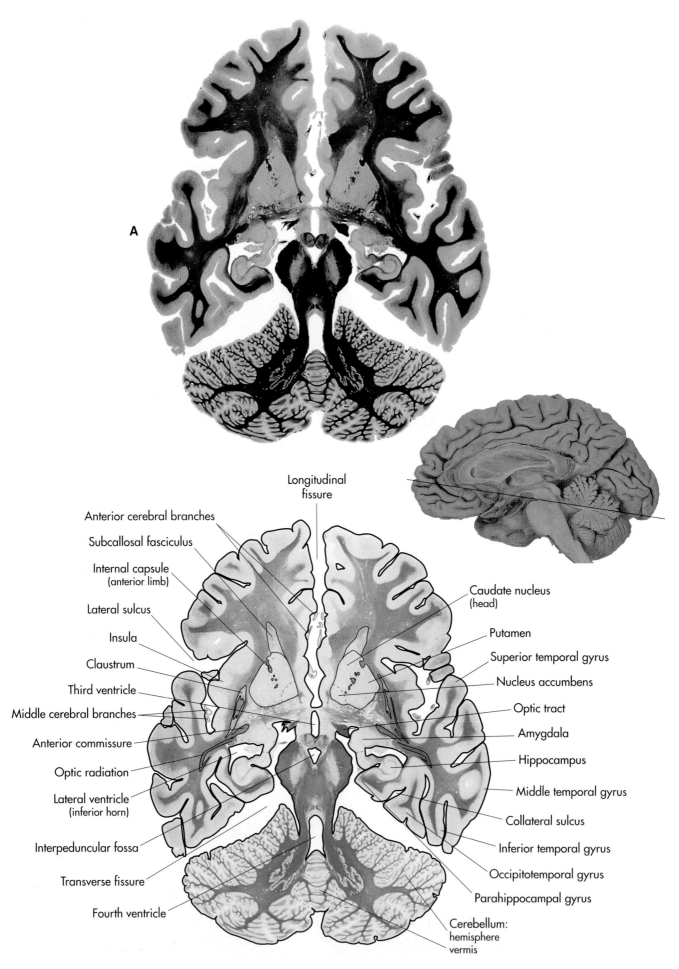

A

Longitudinal
fissure

Anterior cerebral branches

Subcallosal fasciculus

Internal capsule
(anterior limb)

Lateral sulcus

Insula

Claustrum

Third ventricle

Middle cerebral branches

Anterior commissure

Optic radiation

Lateral ventricle
(inferior horn)

Interpeduncular fossa

Transverse fissure

Fourth ventricle

Caudate nucleus
(head)

Putamen

Superior temporal gyrus

Nucleus accumbens

Optic tract

Amygdala

Hippocampus

Middle temporal gyrus

Collateral sulcus

Inferior temporal gyrus

Occipitotemporal gyrus

Parahippocampal gyrus

Cerebellum:
hemisphere
vermis

FIGURE 6-5, cont'd.
B, The central region of Figure 6-5, *A,* enlarged to 1.5× actual size.

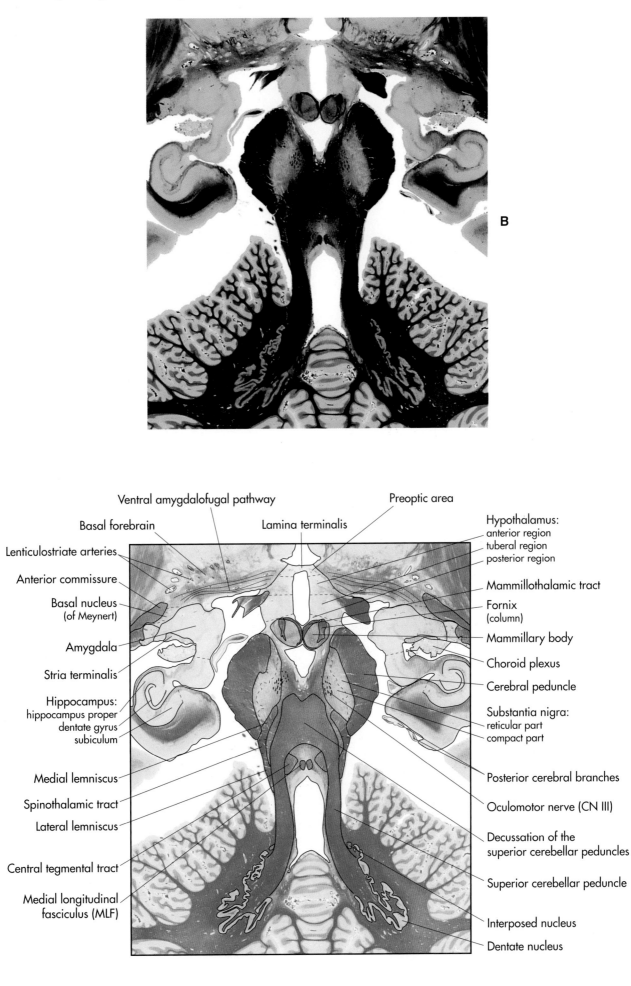

Ventral amygdalofugal pathway

Basal forebrain

Lamina terminalis

Preoptic area

Hypothalamus:
anterior region
tuberal region
posterior region

Lenticulostriate arteries

Anterior commissure

Mammillothalamic tract

Basal nucleus
(of Meynert)

Fornix
(column)

Amygdala

Mammillary body

Stria terminalis

Choroid plexus

Cerebral peduncle

Hippocampus:
hippocampus proper
dentate gyrus
subiculum

Substantia nigra:
reticular part
compact part

Medial lemniscus

Posterior cerebral branches

Spinothalamic tract

Oculomotor nerve (CN III)

Lateral lemniscus

Decussation of the
superior cerebellar peduncles

Central tegmental tract

Superior cerebellar peduncle

Medial longitudinal
fasciculus (MLF)

Interposed nucleus

Dentate nucleus

B

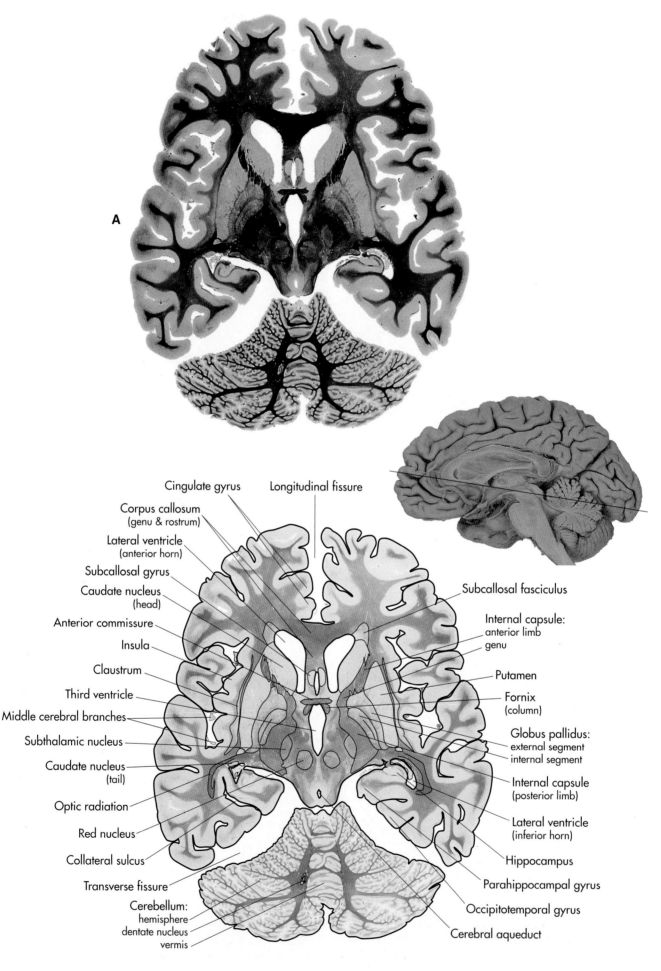

FIGURE 6-6

A, A horizontal section through the anterior commissure. Three fourths actual size.

Cingulate gyrus

Longitudinal fissure

Corpus callosum
(genu & rostrum)

Lateral ventricle
(anterior horn)

Subcallosal gyrus

Caudate nucleus
(head)

Anterior commissure

Insula

Claustrum

Third ventricle

Middle cerebral branches

Subthalamic nucleus

Caudate nucleus
(tail)

Optic radiation

Red nucleus

Collateral sulcus

Transverse fissure

Cerebellum:
hemisphere
dentate nucleus
vermis

Subcallosal fasciculus

Internal capsule:
anterior limb
genu

Putamen

Fornix
(column)

Globus pallidus:
external segment
internal segment

Internal capsule
(posterior limb)

Lateral ventricle
(inferior horn)

Hippocampus

Parahippocampal gyrus

Occipitotemporal gyrus

Cerebral aqueduct

FIGURE 6-6, cont'd.
B, The central region of Figure 6-6, *A,* enlarged to 1.5× actual size.

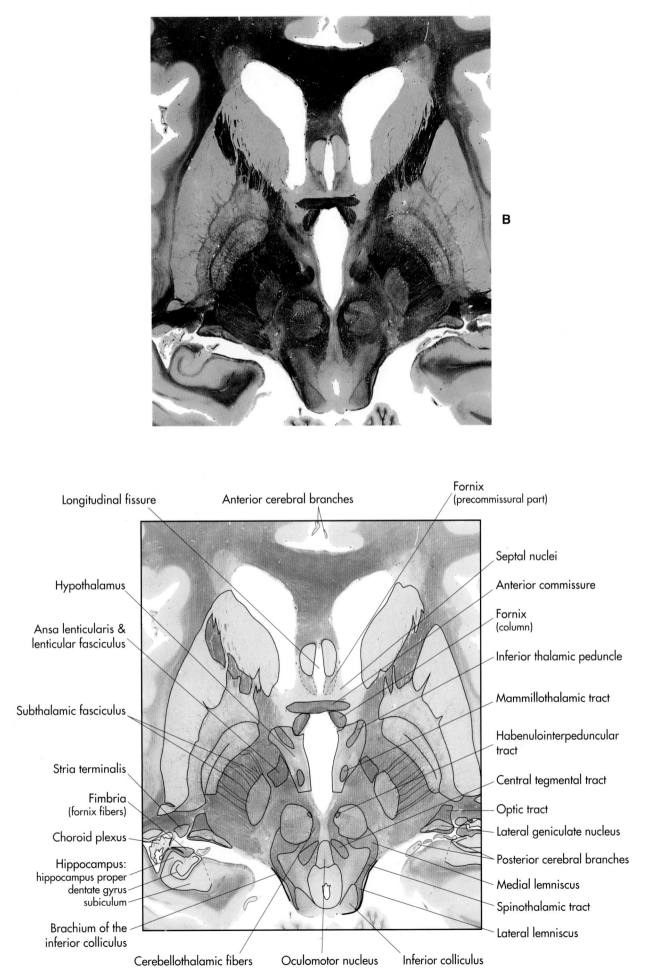

B

Longitudinal fissure

Anterior cerebral branches

Fornix
(precommissural part)

Hypothalamus

Septal nuclei

Anterior commissure

Ansa lenticularis &
lenticular fasciculus

Fornix
(column)

Inferior thalamic peduncle

Subthalamic fasciculus

Mammillothalamic tract

Habenulointerpeduncular
tract

Stria terminalis

Central tegmental tract

Fimbria
(fornix fibers)

Optic tract

Lateral geniculate nucleus

Choroid plexus

Posterior cerebral branches

Hippocampus:
hippocampus proper
dentate gyrus
subiculum

Medial lemniscus

Spinothalamic tract

Brachium of the
inferior colliculus

Lateral lemniscus

Cerebellothalamic fibers

Oculomotor nucleus

Inferior colliculus

FIGURE 6-7
A, A horizontal section through the interventricular foramen and posterior commissure. Three fourths actual size.

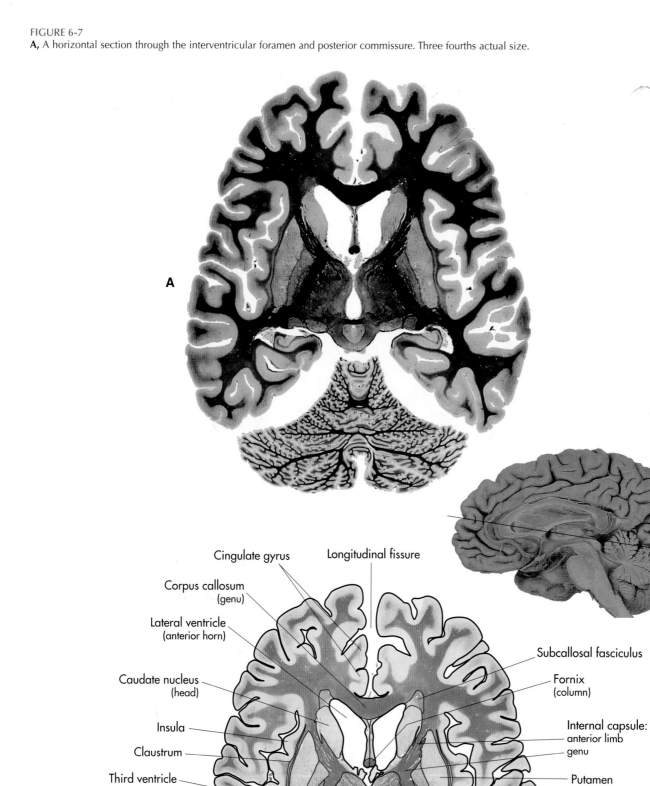

Cingulate gyrus

Longitudinal fissure

Corpus callosum
(genu)

Lateral ventricle
(anterior horn)

Caudate nucleus
(head)

Insula

Claustrum

Third ventricle

Middle cerebral branch

Caudate nucleus
(tail)

Optic radiation

Collateral sulcus

Transverse fissure

Cerebellum:
  hemisphere
  vermis

Subcallosal fasciculus

Fornix
(column)

Internal capsule:
  anterior limb
  genu

Putamen

Globus pallidus
(external segment)

Internal capsule:
  posterior limb
  retrolenticular part

Lateral ventricle
(inferior horn)

Hippocampus

Parahippocampal gyrus

Cerebral aqueduct

FIGURE 6-7, cont'd.
B, The central region of Figure 6-7, *A,* enlarged to 1.5× actual size.

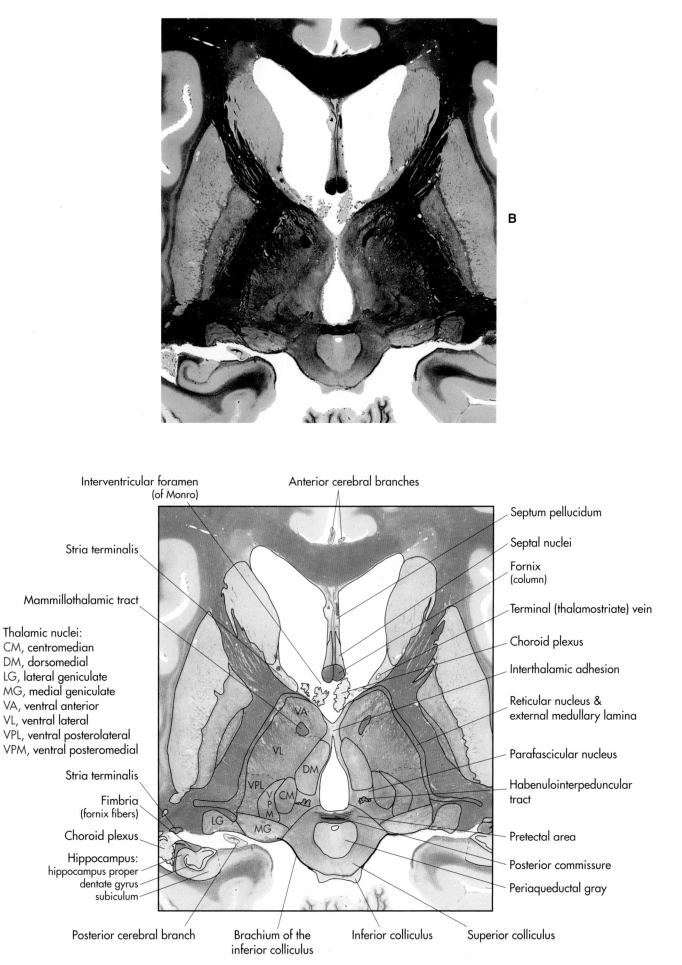

B

Interventricular foramen
(of Monro)

Anterior cerebral branches

Stria terminalis

Septum pellucidum

Septal nuclei

Mammillothalamic tract

Fornix
(column)

Thalamic nuclei:
CM, centromedian
DM, dorsomedial
LG, lateral geniculate
MG, medial geniculate
VA, ventral anterior
VL, ventral lateral
VPL, ventral posterolateral
VPM, ventral posteromedial

Terminal (thalamostriate) vein

Choroid plexus

Interthalamic adhesion

Reticular nucleus &
external medullary lamina

Parafascicular nucleus

Stria terminalis

Habenulointerpeduncular
tract

Fimbria
(fornix fibers)

Choroid plexus

Pretectal area

Hippocampus:
hippocampus proper
dentate gyrus
subiculum

Posterior commissure

Periaqueductal gray

Posterior cerebral branch

Brachium of the
inferior colliculus

Inferior colliculus

Superior colliculus

FIGURE 6-8
A, A horizontal section through the midthalamus. Three fourths actual size.

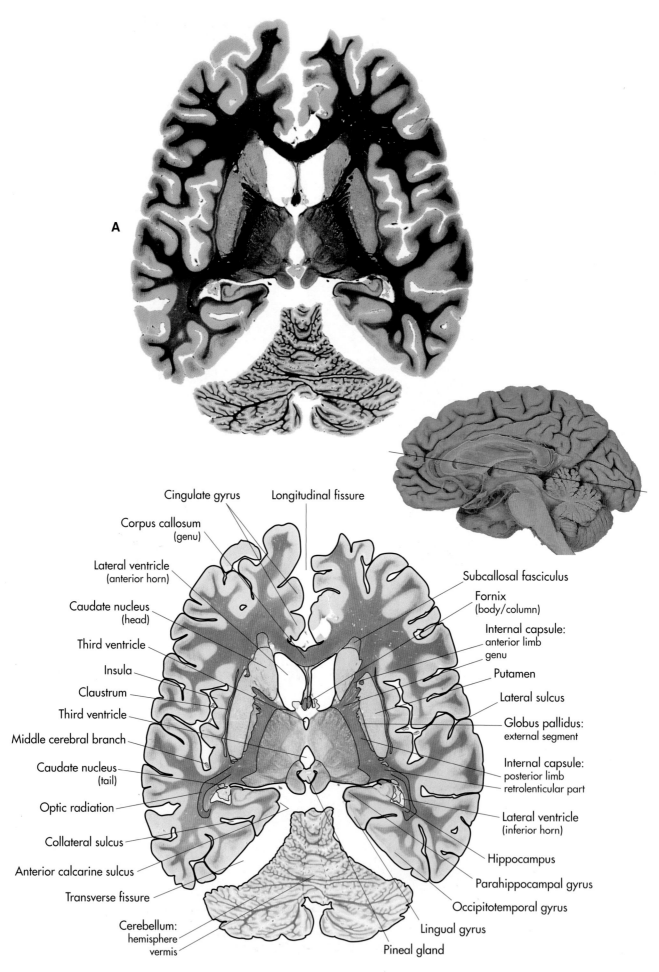

Cingulate gyrus

Longitudinal fissure

Corpus callosum
(genu)

Lateral ventricle
(anterior horn)

Caudate nucleus
(head)

Third ventricle

Insula

Claustrum

Third ventricle

Middle cerebral branch

Caudate nucleus
(tail)

Optic radiation

Collateral sulcus

Anterior calcarine sulcus

Transverse fissure

Cerebellum:
hemisphere
vermis

Subcallosal fasciculus

Fornix
(body/column)

Internal capsule:
anterior limb
genu

Putamen

Lateral sulcus

Globus pallidus:
external segment

Internal capsule:
posterior limb
retrolenticular part

Lateral ventricle
(inferior horn)

Hippocampus

Parahippocampal gyrus

Occipitotemporal gyrus

Lingual gyrus

Pineal gland

FIGURE 6-8, cont'd.
B, The central region of Figure 6-8, *A,* enlarged to 1.5× actual size.

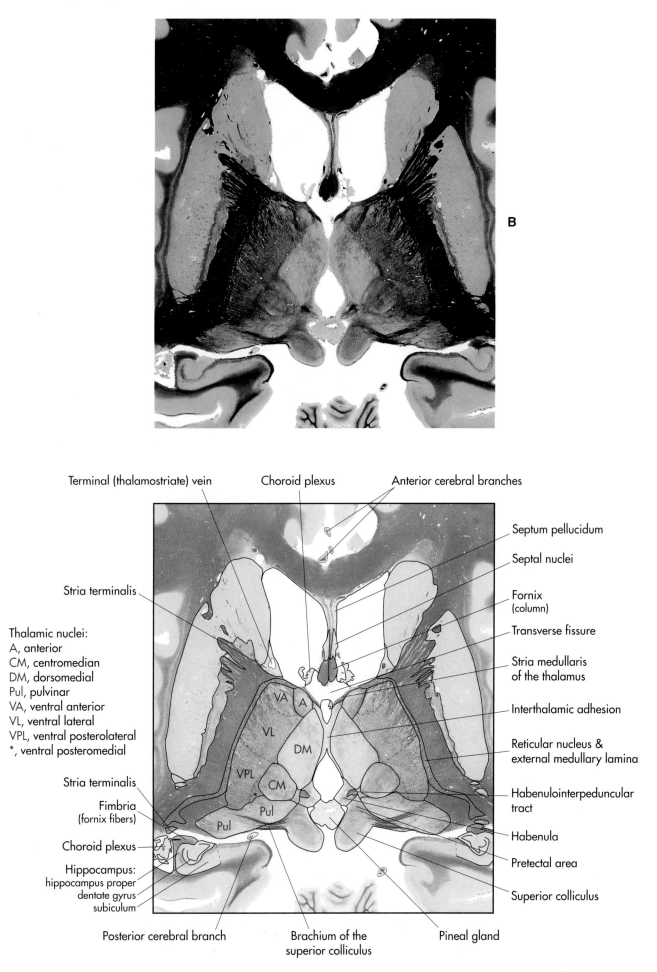

B

Terminal (thalamostriate) vein

Choroid plexus

Anterior cerebral branches

Stria terminalis

Thalamic nuclei:
A, anterior
CM, centromedian
DM, dorsomedial
Pul, pulvinar
VA, ventral anterior
VL, ventral lateral
VPL, ventral posterolateral
*, ventral posteromedial

Stria terminalis

Fimbria
(fornix fibers)

Choroid plexus

Hippocampus:
hippocampus proper
dentate gyrus
subiculum

Septum pellucidum

Septal nuclei

Fornix
(column)

Transverse fissure

Stria medullaris
of the thalamus

Interthalamic adhesion

Reticular nucleus &
external medullary lamina

Habenulointerpeduncular
tract

Habenula

Pretectal area

Superior colliculus

VA A

VL

DM

VPL

CM

*

Pul

Pul

Posterior cerebral branch

Brachium of the
superior colliculus

Pineal gland

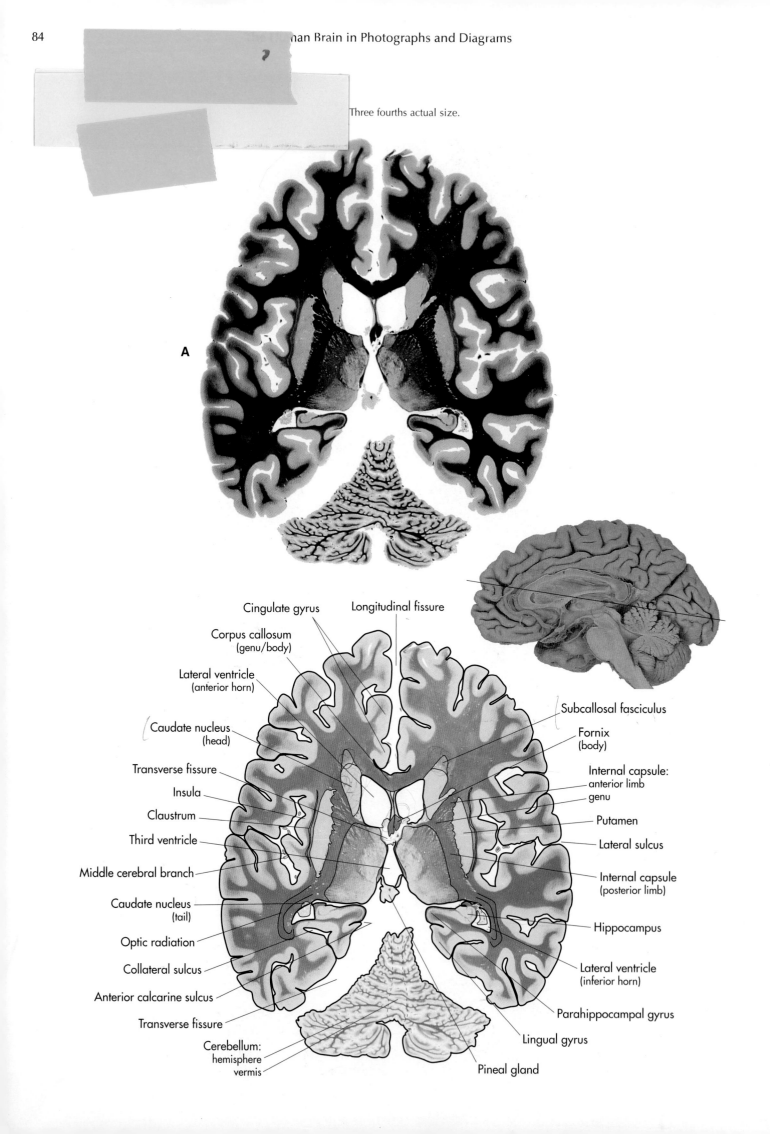

Three fourths actual size.

A

Cingulate gyrus

Longitudinal fissure

Corpus callosum
(genu/body)

Lateral ventricle
(anterior horn)

Subcallosal fasciculus

Caudate nucleus
(head)

Fornix
(body)

Transverse fissure

Internal capsule:
anterior limb
genu

Insula

Claustrum

Putamen

Third ventricle

Lateral sulcus

Middle cerebral branch

Internal capsule
(posterior limb)

Caudate nucleus
(tail)

Hippocampus

Optic radiation

Collateral sulcus

Lateral ventricle
(inferior horn)

Anterior calcarine sulcus

Parahippocampal gyrus

Transverse fissure

Lingual gyrus

Cerebellum:
hemisphere
vermis

Pineal gland

FIGURE 6-9, cont'd.
B, The central region of Figure 6-9, *A,* enlarged to 1.5× actual size.

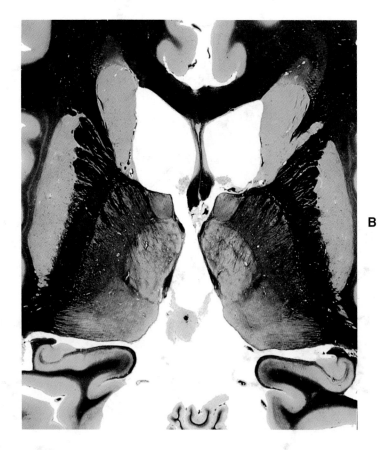

B

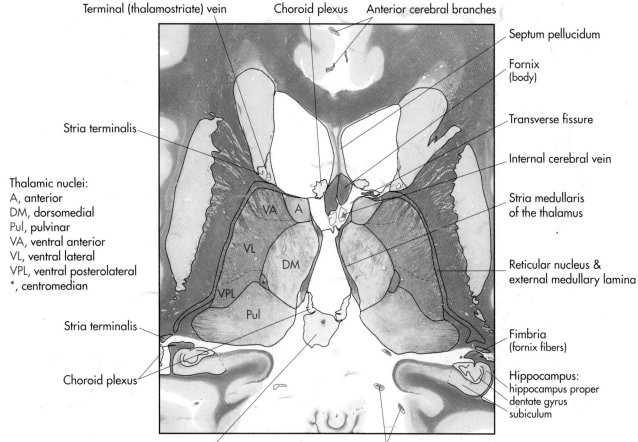

Terminal (thalamostriate) vein

Choroid plexus

Anterior cerebral branches

Septum pellucidum

Fornix
(body)

Transverse fissure

Internal cerebral vein

Stria medullaris
of the thalamus

Reticular nucleus &
external medullary lamina

Fimbria
(fornix fibers)

Hippocampus:
hippocampus proper
dentate gyrus
subiculum

Stria terminalis

Thalamic nuclei:
A, anterior
DM, dorsomedial
Pul, pulvinar
VA, ventral anterior
VL, ventral lateral
VPL, ventral posterolateral
*, centromedian

VA A

VL

DM

VPL

*

Pul

Stria terminalis

Choroid plexus

Pineal gland

Posterior cerebral branches

FIGURE 6-10
A, A horizontal section through the transverse fissure and internal cerebral veins. Three fourths actual size.

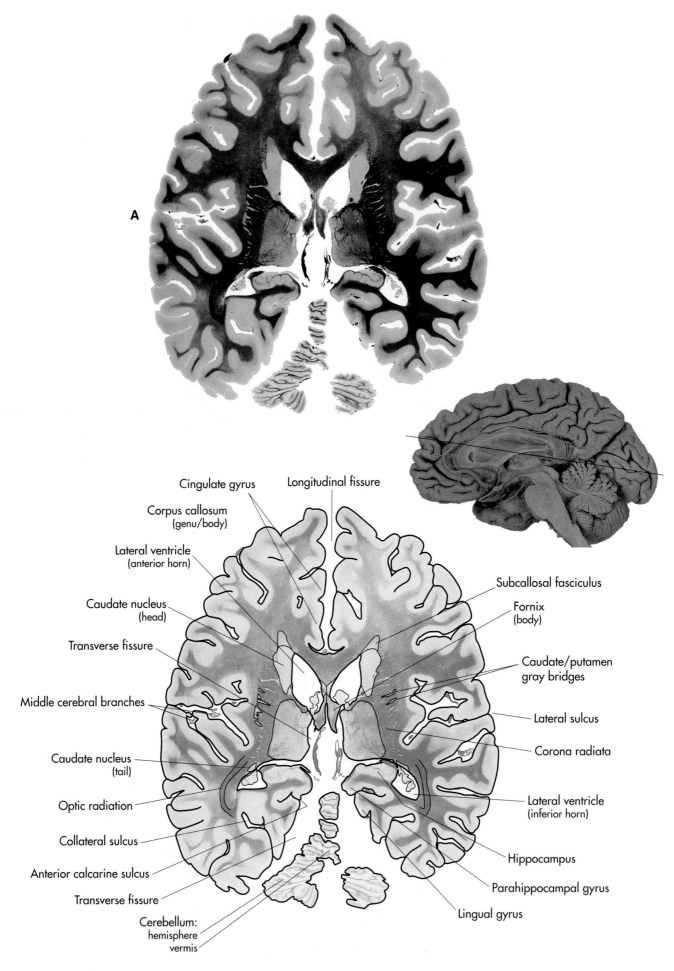

Cingulate gyrus

Longitudinal fissure

Corpus callosum
(genu/body)

Lateral ventricle
(anterior horn)

Caudate nucleus
(head)

Transverse fissure

Middle cerebral branches

Caudate nucleus
(tail)

Optic radiation

Collateral sulcus

Anterior calcarine sulcus

Transverse fissure

Cerebellum:
hemisphere
vermis

Subcallosal fasciculus

Fornix
(body)

Caudate/putamen
gray bridges

Lateral sulcus

Corona radiata

Lateral ventricle
(inferior horn)

Hippocampus

Parahippocampal gyrus

Lingual gyrus

FIGURE 6-10, cont'd.
B, The central region of Figure 6-10, *A,* enlarged to 1.5× actual size.

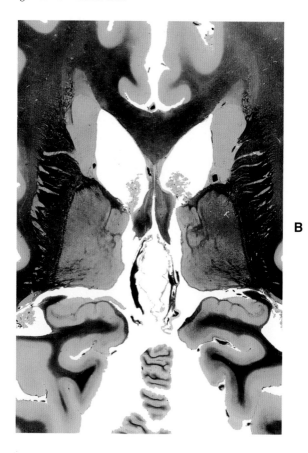

B

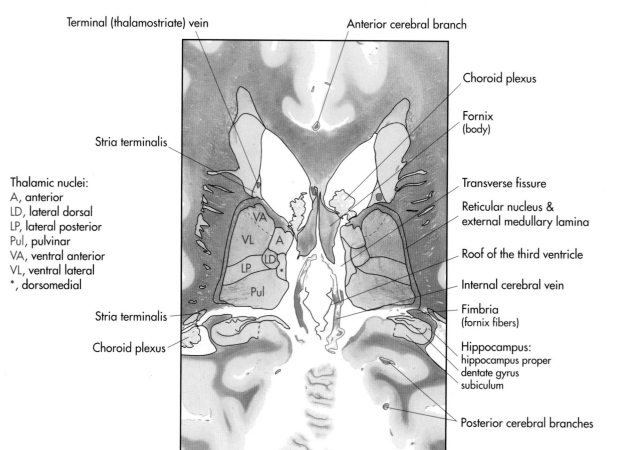

Terminal (thalamostriate) vein

Anterior cerebral branch

Choroid plexus

Fornix
(body)

Stria terminalis

Thalamic nuclei:
A, anterior
LD, lateral dorsal
LP, lateral posterior
Pul, pulvinar
VA, ventral anterior
VL, ventral lateral
*, dorsomedial

Transverse fissure

Reticular nucleus &
external medullary lamina

Roof of the third ventricle

Internal cerebral vein

Stria terminalis

Fimbria
(fornix fibers)

Choroid plexus

Hippocampus:
hippocampus proper
dentate gyrus
subiculum

Posterior cerebral branches

VA
VL
A
LD
LP
*
Pul

SAGITTAL SECTIONS

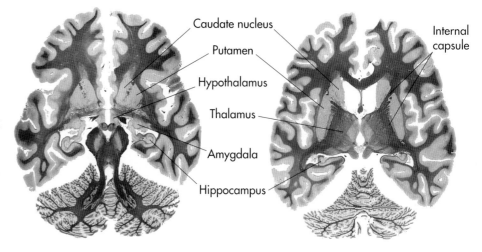

This chapter, the last of three showing sections of entire human brains, illustrates parasagittal planes. Forebrain structures continue to be emphasized, but parts of the brainstem and cerebellum are indicated as well. The organization of various functional systems in the forebrain (e.g., thalamus, hippocampus) is presented in Chapter 8.

FIGURE 7-1
The horizontal sections from Figures 6-3, *G* and *N,* used in much of this chapter to indicate planes of section.

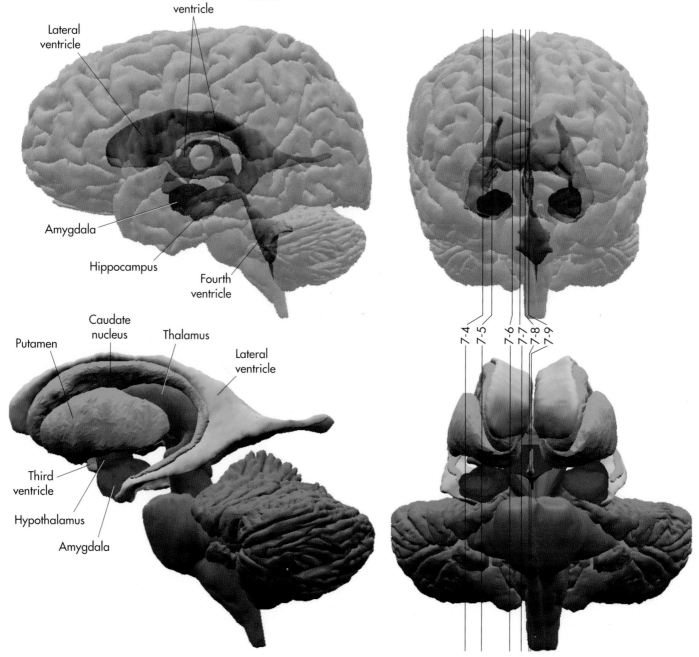

FIGURE 7-2
The planes of section shown in this chapter, indicated on three-dimensional reconstructions. *(Courtesy of Dr. John W. Sundsten, Department of Biological Structure, University of Washington School of Medicine.)*

FIGURE 7-3

Sixteen sagittal sections of the right hemisphere of a brain. The sections are arranged in a lateral-to-medial sequence extending from the insula to the midline. Anterior is toward the left, so the view is as though you were backing through the brain, always looking from inside the brain out toward the lateral sulcus.

A, The first section passes tangentially through the insula (5) and shows nicely how the lateral sulcus (6) leads to it and the circular sulcus (4) outlines it. The precentral (1) and postcentral (3) gyri can also be seen, separated from each other by the central sulcus (2), which, cut obliquely, seems deeper than it really is.

B, The circular sulcus (1) is still present, partially surrounding the insula (2), but now the plane of section begins to reveal structures just deep to insular cortex—in this case the claustrum (3, 6). The most lateral part of the lateral ventricle, the inferior horn (5), also appears, with the tail of the caudate nucleus (4) cut tangentially in its wall.

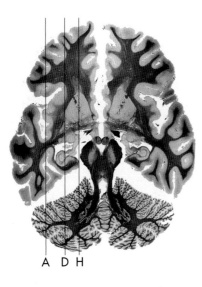

C, Now the putamen (1) appears and the claustrum (5), a sheet of gray matter that covers the curved lateral aspect of the putamen, appears to partially surround it in this two-dimensional view. The tail of the caudate nucleus (2) is cut tangentially in the wall of the inferior horn of the lateral ventricle (3). Across the ventricle, the hippocampus (4) makes its appearance.

D, The putamen (1) continues to increase in size, still partially surrounded by the claustrum (9). The tail of the caudate nucleus (2, 6) is now cut in two places as it curves into the temporal lobe with the inferior horn of the lateral ventricle (5). The posterior horn of the lateral ventricle (3) extends back toward the occipital lobe. The hippocampus (4) increases in size, and the amygdala (7) appears at its anterior end. A downward extension (8) of the putamen merges with the amygdala, much as the tail of the caudate nucleus merges with both in a nearby plane (see Figure 7-3, E). Fibers that have collected from the temporal lobe and will cross in the anterior commissure (10) mass underneath the putamen.

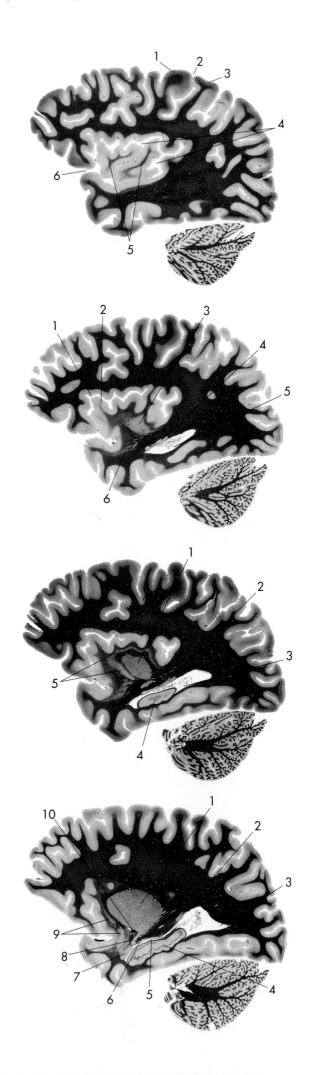

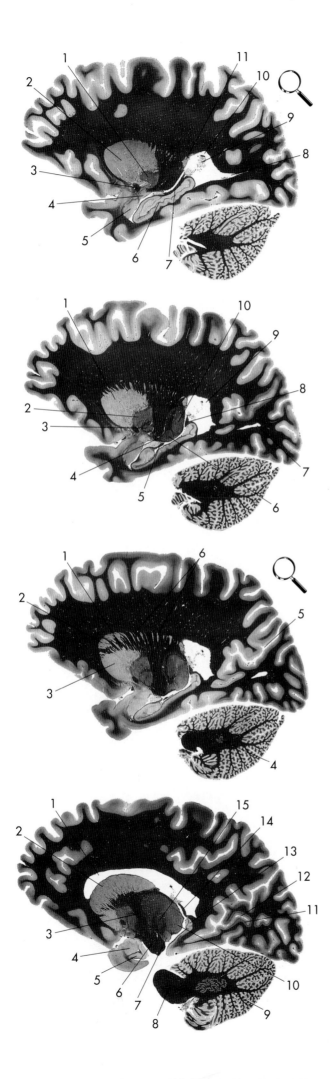

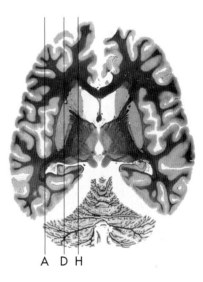

FIGURE 7-3, cont'd.
Sagittal sections.

E, The globus pallidus (1, part of its external segment) appears adjacent to the putamen (2), with fibers of the anterior commissure (3) traveling beneath them. The caudate nucleus is again cut twice, once (11) as it curves around from the body to the inferior horn of the lateral ventricle and a second time (4) as it merges with the amygdala (5). Fibers of the fimbria (7) are cut tangentially as they emerge from the hippocampus (6). An enlarged mass of choroid plexus (9, the glomus) protrudes into the atrium of the lateral ventricle (10) and the posterior horn of the ventricle (8) extends back into the occipital lobe. Shown enlarged in Figure 7-4.

F, Now both the internal (3) and external (2) segments of the globus pallidus can be seen adjacent to the putamen (1). The plane of section has reached the thalamus—the pulvinar (10) appears, as well as the lateral geniculate nucleus (6) with the optic tract (4) ending in it. The fimbria, cut tangentially in Figure 7-3, E, is now cut in two places (5, 8). The posterior horn of the lateral ventricle (7) appears in this plane to be a detached cavity in the occipital lobe, but is in fact continuous with the atrium (9).

G, The head of the caudate nucleus (2) appears, with fibers of the anterior limb of the internal capsule (1) emerging from the cleft between it and the putamen (3). Strands of gray matter (6) extend between the caudate nucleus and putamen, emphasizing the common embryological origin and similar pattern of connections of these two parts of the striatum. The most lateral of the deep cerebellar nuclei, the dentate nucleus (4), can be seen, and the parietooccipital sulcus (5) is now distinct. Shown enlarged in Figure 7-5.

H, The head of the caudate nucleus (2) is cut tangentially in the wall of the anterior horn of the lateral ventricle (1). The continuity between the internal capsule (3, here the genu) and cerebral peduncle (6) is apparent. In the temporal lobe, the amygdala (4) and the anterior end of the hippocampus (5) underlie the uncus, and the fimbria is in the process of separating from the most caudal bit of hippocampus (13) and continuing as the crus of the fornix (14). The plane of section has moved deeper into the thalamus and the medial geniculate nucleus (7), pulvinar (10), and nuclei of the lateral division (15, here VPL) can be seen. The dentate nucleus (9) is more fully formed, and visual cortex (11) forms the banks of the calcarine sulcus (12). The middle cerebellar peduncle (8) leaves the basal pons and enters the cerebellum.

FIGURE 7-3, cont'd.
Sagittal sections.

I, As the plane of section moves medially, progressively more of the prominent sulci of the medial surface of the brain become apparent—in this case the cingulate sulcus *(1)* and its marginal branch *(2)*. The subthalamic nucleus *(4)* and substantia nigra *(5)* appear beneath the thalamus, and the continuous white-matter path from the internal capsule *(3)* through the cerebral peduncle *(6)* and into the basal pons *(7)* is shown nicely. The optic tract *(8)* proceeds posteriorly toward the lateral geniculate nucleus and fibers of the anterior commissure *(9)* proceed toward (or away from) the midline.

J, The subthalamic nucleus *(3)* and substantia nigra *(4)* are still apparent, and the centromedian nucleus *(1)* can now be seen in the thalamus. Fibers that formed the fimbria in previous sections of this series are now separated from the hippocampus and proceeding anteriorly as the crus of the fornix *(2)*. The inferior cerebellar peduncle *(5)* turns dorsally and enters the cerebellum. The uncus *(6)* appears for the last time. Shown enlarged in Figure 7-6.

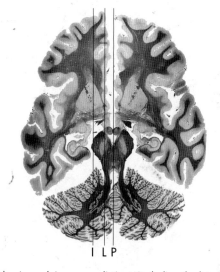

K, Many thalamic nuclei are now distinct, including the lateral dorsal *(1)*, dorsomedial *(2)*, centromedian *(3)*, pulvinar *(4)*, ventral anterior *(14)*, ventral lateral *(15)* and anterior *(16)*. The olfactory tract *(13)* moves posteriorly across the orbital surface of the frontal lobe. As the plane of section approaches the midline, more brainstem components begin to become apparent, including the superior *(7)* and inferior *(8)* colliculi and the red nucleus *(12)*, adjacent to the substantia nigra *(11)*. The superior cerebellar peduncle *(10)* emerges from the cerebellum and the interposed nucleus *(9)* largely replaces the dentate nucleus. Visual cortex *(5)* lines the calcarine sulcus *(6)*.

L, Now the anterior nucleus *(1)* of the thalamus enlarges, with the mammillothalamic tract *(3)* ascending into it. The fornix is cut nearly tangentially through the crus *(2)*. Fibers of the anterior commissure *(13)* continue on their course toward the midline, and the right optic nerve *(11)* proceeds into the optic chiasm *(10)*. Brainstem structures that can be seen more clearly or for the first time include the red nucleus *(4)*, superior cerebellar peduncle *(5)*, fourth ventricle *(6)*, inferior olivary nucleus *(7)*, and the pyramid *(8)* emerging from the basal pons *(9)*. Nucleus accumbens *(12)* can be seen near the base of the forebrain, in continuity with the head of the caudate nucleus *(14)*. Shown enlarged in Figure 7-7.

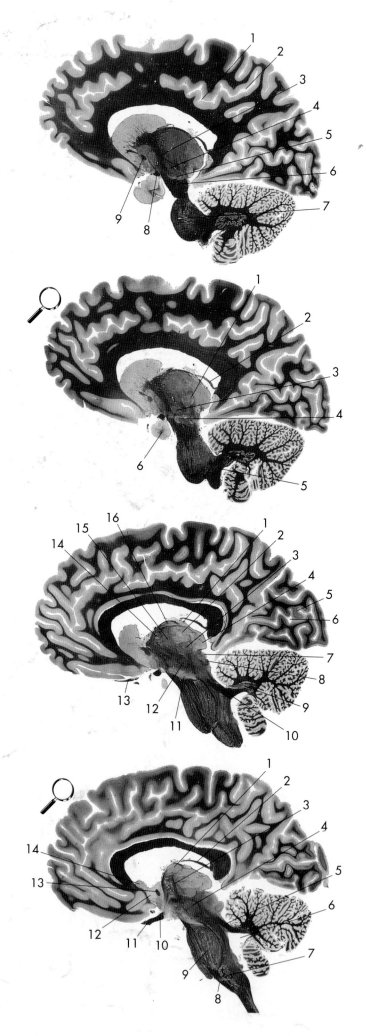

FIGURE 7-3, cont'd.
Sagittal sections.

M, The fornix is cut twice (although nearly tangentially in each instance)—through the crus and body *(1)* and as the column *(4)* ends in the mammillary body *(7),* from which the mammillothalamic tract *(2)* emanates. The physical continuity between the septal nuclei *(3)* and the hypothalamus *(5)* is apparent. The cingulate gyrus *(16)* narrows into an isthmus *(13)* through which it is continuous with the parahippocampal gyrus. Half the fibers from each optic nerve cross the midline in the optic chiasm *(6),* and the habenulointerpeduncular tract *(14)* descends from the habenula *(15).* Brainstem and cerebellar structures include the superior and inferior colliculi *(12),* periaqueductal gray *(10),* fastigial nucleus *(11),* and fibers of the superior cerebellar peduncle that emerge from their decussation *(9)* and pass through or around the red nucleus *(8).*

N, The plane of section, now very near the midline, passes through the body *(1)* and column *(2)* of the fornix as the latter travels just behind the anterior commissure *(3).* The hypothalamus *(4),* including the mammillary body *(5)* and emerging mammillothalamic fibers *(7),* forms the wall and floor of the third ventricle. Other near-midline structures include the basilar artery *(6),* pineal gland *(8),* and great cerebral vein of Galen *(9).* Shown enlarged in Figure 7-8.

O, All the parts of the corpus callosum—the body *(1),* genu *(4),* rostrum *(6),* and splenium *(12)*—are now apparent. The septum pellucidum *(3)* merges with the septal nuclei *(5),* the fornix *(2)* is once again cut tangentially, and choroid plexus *(7)* passes through the interventricular foramen. The stria medullaris of the thalamus *(13)* proceeds posteriorly toward the habenula. Brainstem structures include the medial longitudinal fasciculus *(11),* the decussating superior cerebellar peduncles *(10),* and their continuation as cerebellothalamic fibers *(8)* surrounding the red nucleus *(9).*

P, Almost exactly in the midline, the internal cerebral vein *(1)* travels posteriorly to join the great cerebral vein of Galen *(10).* Much of the ventricular system can also be seen, including the cerebral aqueduct *(7)* and the fourth ventricle *(8).* The section did not quite follow the entire septum pellucidum, and part of the anterior horn of the lateral ventricle *(2)* is visible through the resulting hole. The third ventricle *(3)* and its parts and boundaries are shown nicely: the lamina terminalis *(4)* at the rostral end of the ventricle, and the optic *(5),* infundibular *(6),* and pineal *(9)* recesses. Shown enlarged in Figure 7-9.

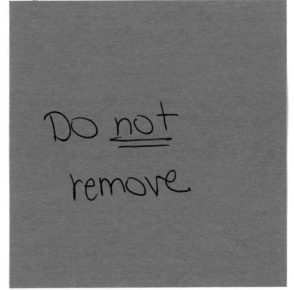

FIGURE 7-4
A, A parasagittal section passing longitudinally through much of the hippocampus. Actual size.

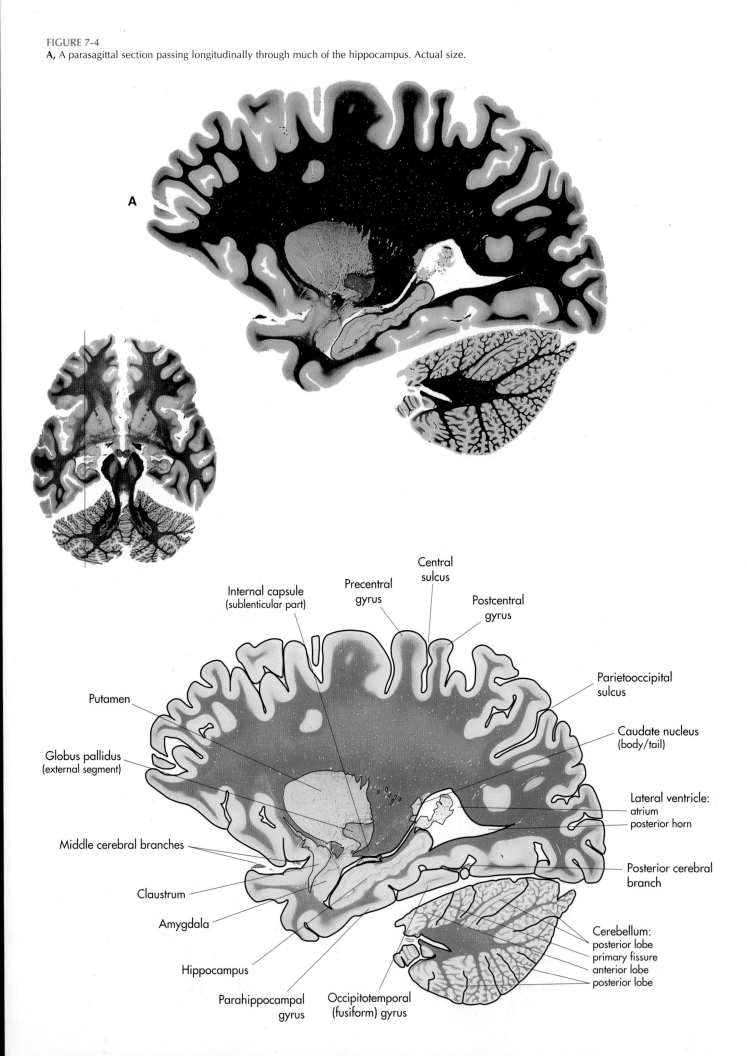

A

Internal capsule
(sublenticular part)

Precentral
gyrus

Central
sulcus

Postcentral
gyrus

Parietooccipital
sulcus

Putamen

Caudate nucleus
(body/tail)

Globus pallidus
(external segment)

Lateral ventricle:
atrium
posterior horn

Middle cerebral branches

Posterior cerebral
branch

Claustrum

Amygdala

Cerebellum:
posterior lobe
primary fissure
anterior lobe
posterior lobe

Hippocampus

Parahippocampal
gyrus

Occipitotemporal
(fusiform) gyrus

FIGURE 7-4, cont'd.
B, The central region of Figure 7-4, *A,* enlarged to 1.7× actual size.

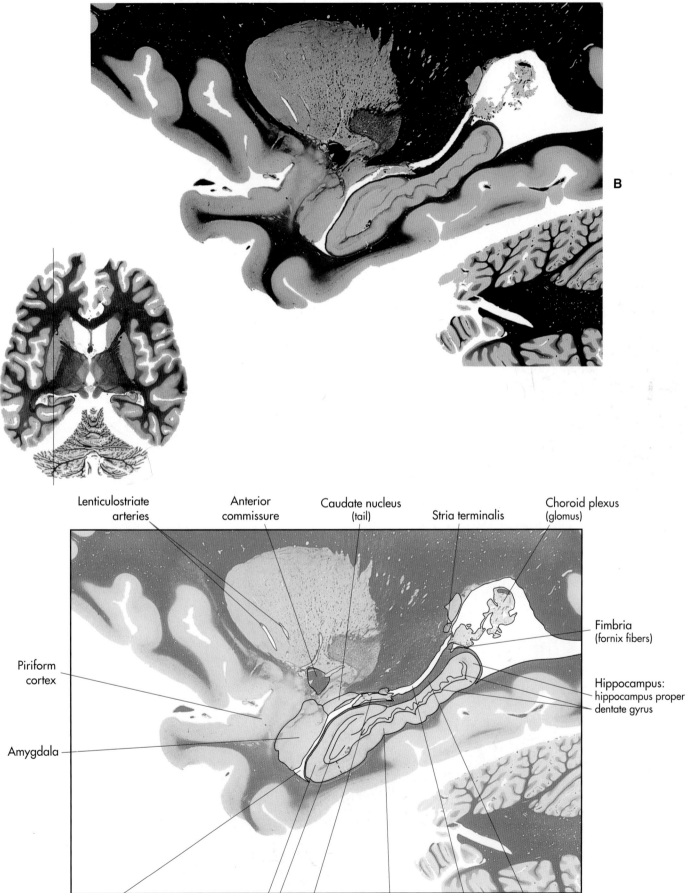

B

Lenticulostriate arteries

Anterior commissure

Caudate nucleus (tail)

Stria terminalis

Choroid plexus (glomus)

Piriform cortex

Fimbria (fornix fibers)

Hippocampus: hippocampus proper dentate gyrus

Amygdala

Lateral ventricle (inferior horn)

Hippocampus: hippocampus proper dentate gyrus

Choroid plexus

Subiculum

Choroid fissure

Fimbria (fornix fibers)

FIGURE 7-5
A, A parasagittal section through the amygdala and hippocampus. Actual size.

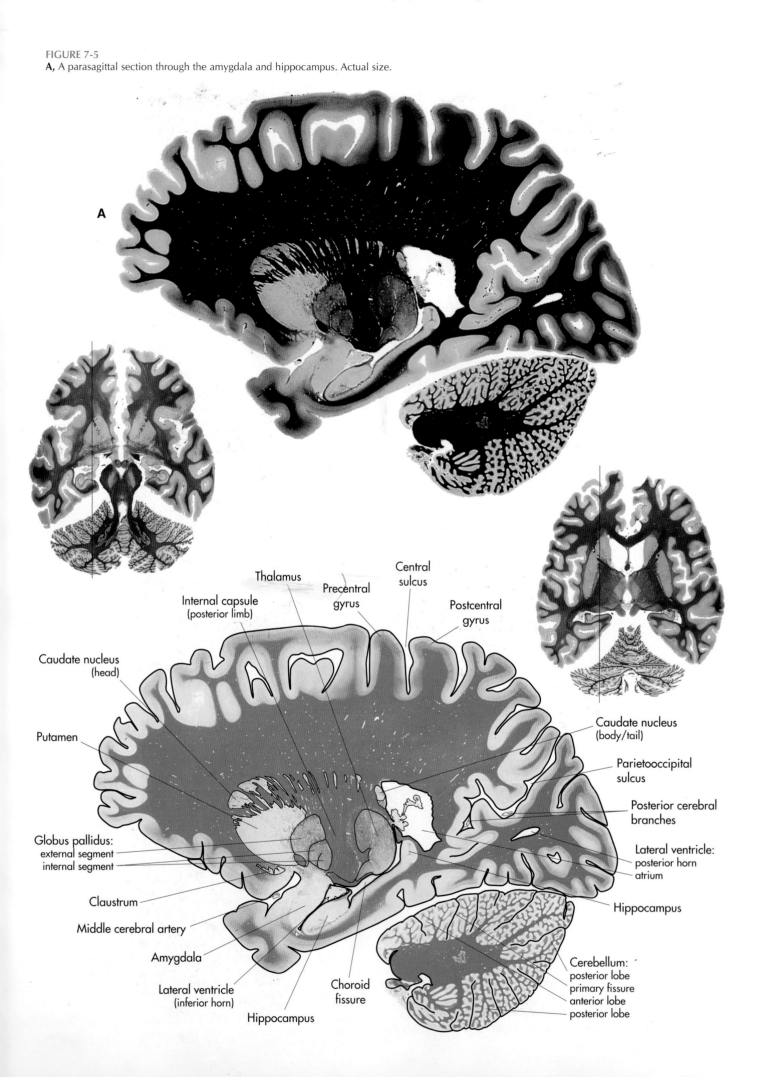

A

Thalamus

Central
sulcus

Internal capsule
(posterior limb)

Precentral
gyrus

Postcentral
gyrus

Caudate nucleus
(head)

Caudate nucleus
(body/tail)

Putamen

Parietooccipital
sulcus

Posterior cerebral
branches

Globus pallidus:
external segment
internal segment

Lateral ventricle:
posterior horn
atrium

Claustrum

Hippocampus

Middle cerebral artery

Amygdala

Cerebellum:
posterior lobe
primary fissure
anterior lobe
posterior lobe

Lateral ventricle
(inferior horn)

Choroid
fissure

Hippocampus

FIGURE 7-5, cont'd.
B, The central region of Figure 7-5, *A,* enlarged to 1.7× actual size.

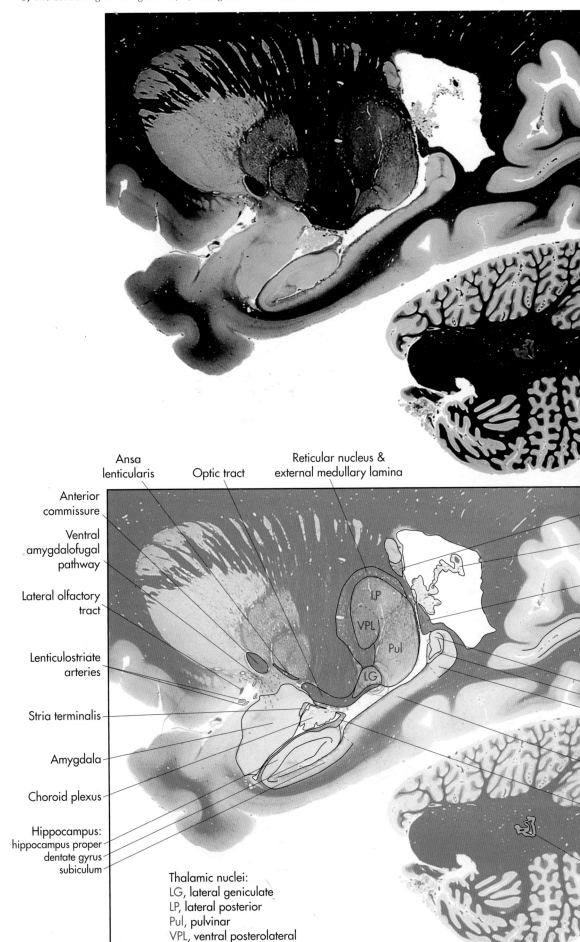

B

Ansa lenticularis

Optic tract

Reticular nucleus & external medullary lamina

Anterior commissure

Ventral amygdalofugal pathway

Lateral olfactory tract

Lenticulostriate arteries

Stria terminalis

Amygdala

Choroid plexus

Hippocampus:
hippocampus proper
dentate gyrus
subiculum

Stria terminalis

Choroid plexus (glomus)

Fimbria (fornix fibers)

Visual cortex (stripe of Gennari)

Hippocampus:
hippocampus proper
dentate gyrus
subiculum

Parahippocampal gyrus

Fimbria (fornix fibers)

Dentate nucleus

LP

VPL

Pul

LG

Thalamic nuclei:
LG, lateral geniculate
LP, lateral posterior
Pul, pulvinar
VPL, ventral posterolateral

FIGURE 7-6
A, A parasagittal section through the uncus and the middle of the thalamus. Actual size.

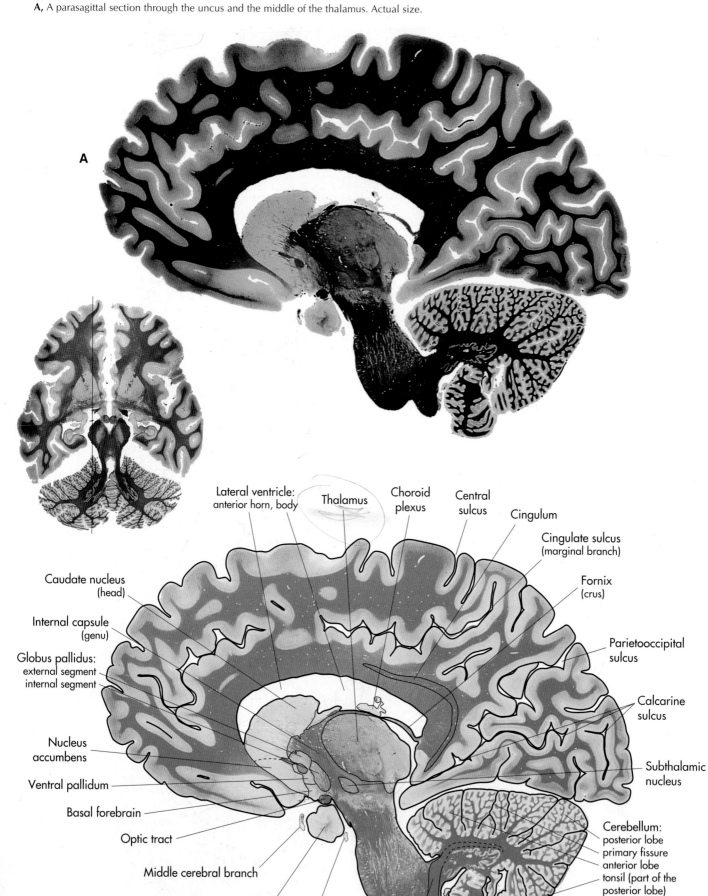

A

Lateral ventricle:
anterior horn, body

Thalamus

Choroid
plexus

Central
sulcus

Cingulum

Cingulate sulcus
(marginal branch)

Caudate nucleus
(head)

Fornix
(crus)

Internal capsule
(genu)

Parietooccipital
sulcus

Globus pallidus:
external segment
internal segment

Calcarine
sulcus

Nucleus
accumbens

Ventral pallidum

Subthalamic
nucleus

Basal forebrain

Cerebellum:
posterior lobe
primary fissure
anterior lobe
tonsil (part of the
posterior lobe)

Optic tract

Middle cerebral branch

Uncus

Posterior cerebral branch

Inferior
cerebellar
peduncle

FIGURE 7-6, cont'd.
B, The central region of Figure 7-6, *A,* enlarged to 1.7× actual size.

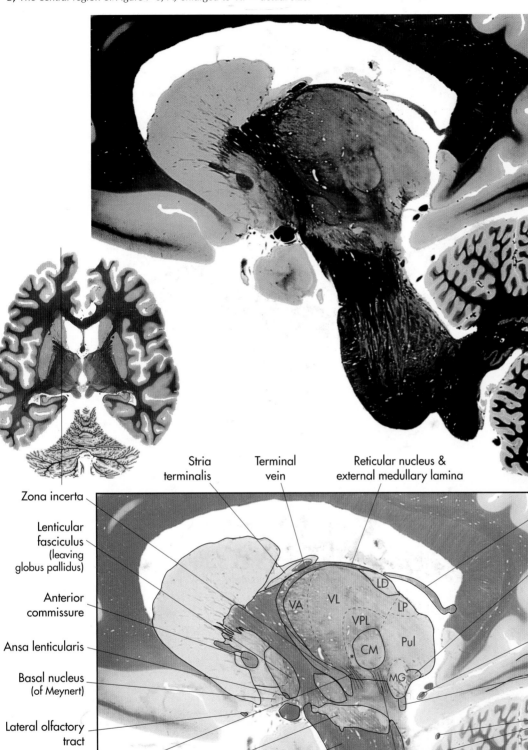

B

Stria
terminalis

Terminal
vein

Reticular nucleus &
external medullary lamina

Fornix
(crus)

Zona incerta

Lenticular
fasciculus
(leaving
globus pallidus)

Anterior
commissure

Ansa lenticularis

Basal nucleus
(of Meynert)

Lateral olfactory
tract

Cerebellothalamic
fibers

Substantia nigra

Cerebral
peduncle

Superior
brachium

Visual cortex
(stripe of Gennari)

Posterior
cerebral
branch

Inferior
brachium

Superior
cerebellar
branches

Dentate
nucleus

Trigeminal
main sensory
nucleus

Dorsal
cochlear
nucleus

Posterior
inferior
cerebellar
branch

LD

VA

VL

LP

VPL

Pul

CM

MG

Thalamic nuclei:
CM, centromedian
LD, lateral dorsal
LP, lateral posterior
MG, medial geniculate
Pul, pulvinar
VA, ventral anterior
VL, ventral lateral
VPL, ventral posterolateral
*, ventral posteromedial

Basal
pons

Medial lemniscus,
spinothalamic tract

FIGURE 7-7
A, A parasagittal section through the mammillothalamic tract. Actual size.

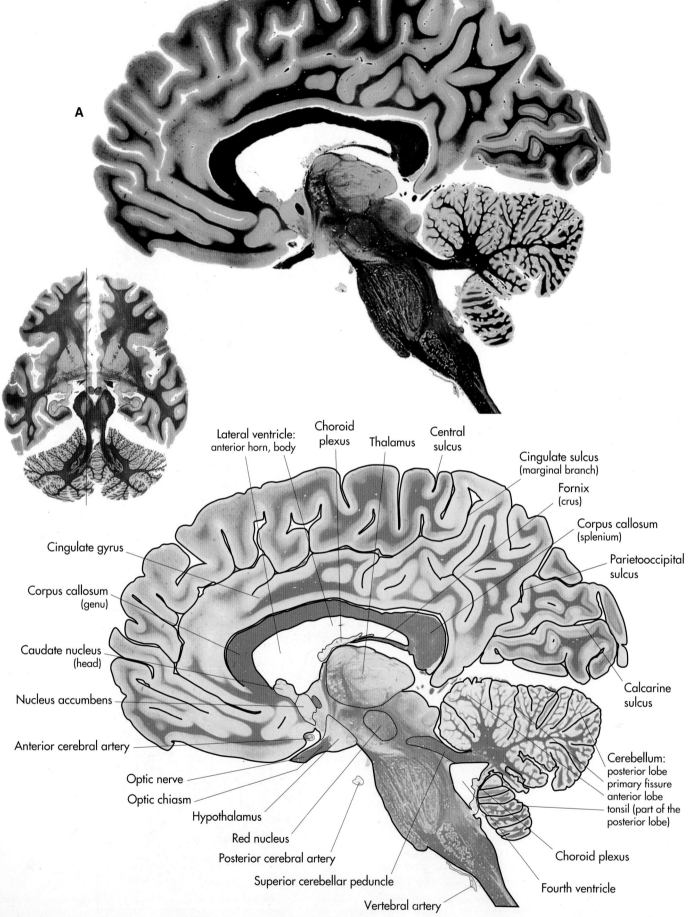

Lateral ventricle: anterior horn, body

Choroid plexus

Thalamus

Central sulcus

Cingulate sulcus (marginal branch)

Fornix (crus)

Corpus callosum (splenium)

Parietooccipital sulcus

Cingulate gyrus

Corpus callosum (genu)

Caudate nucleus (head)

Nucleus accumbens

Anterior cerebral artery

Optic nerve

Optic chiasm

Hypothalamus

Red nucleus

Posterior cerebral artery

Superior cerebellar peduncle

Vertebral artery

Calcarine sulcus

Cerebellum: posterior lobe primary fissure anterior lobe tonsil (part of the posterior lobe)

Choroid plexus

Fourth ventricle

FIGURE 7-7, cont'd.
B, The central region of Figure 7-7, *A,* enlarged to 1.7× actual size.

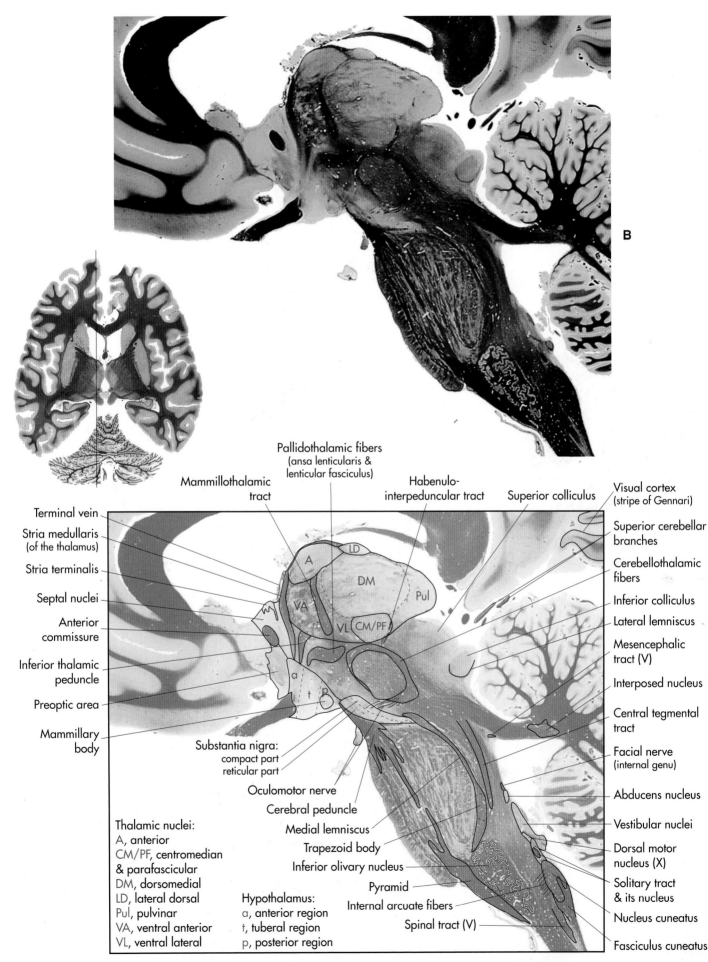

B

Pallidothalamic fibers
(ansa lenticularis &
lenticular fasciculus)

Mammillothalamic
tract

Habenulo-
interpeduncular tract

Superior colliculus

Visual cortex
(stripe of Gennari)

Terminal vein

Stria medullaris
(of the thalamus)

Stria terminalis

Septal nuclei

Anterior
commissure

Inferior thalamic
peduncle

Preoptic area

Mammillary
body

Superior cerebellar
branches

Cerebellothalamic
fibers

Inferior colliculus

Lateral lemniscus

Mesencephalic
tract (V)

Interposed nucleus

Central tegmental
tract

Facial nerve
(internal genu)

Abducens nucleus

Vestibular nuclei

Dorsal motor
nucleus (X)

Solitary tract
& its nucleus

Nucleus cuneatus

Fasciculus cuneatus

A
LD
DM
Pul
VA
VL
CM/PF
a
t p

Substantia nigra:
compact part
reticular part

Oculomotor nerve

Cerebral peduncle

Medial lemniscus

Trapezoid body

Inferior olivary nucleus

Pyramid

Internal arcuate fibers

Spinal tract (V)

Thalamic nuclei:
A, anterior
CM/PF, centromedian
& parafascicular
DM, dorsomedial
LD, lateral dorsal
Pul, pulvinar
VA, ventral anterior
VL, ventral lateral

Hypothalamus:
a, anterior region
t, tuberal region
p, posterior region

FIGURE 7-8
A, A parasagittal section near the midline. Actual size.

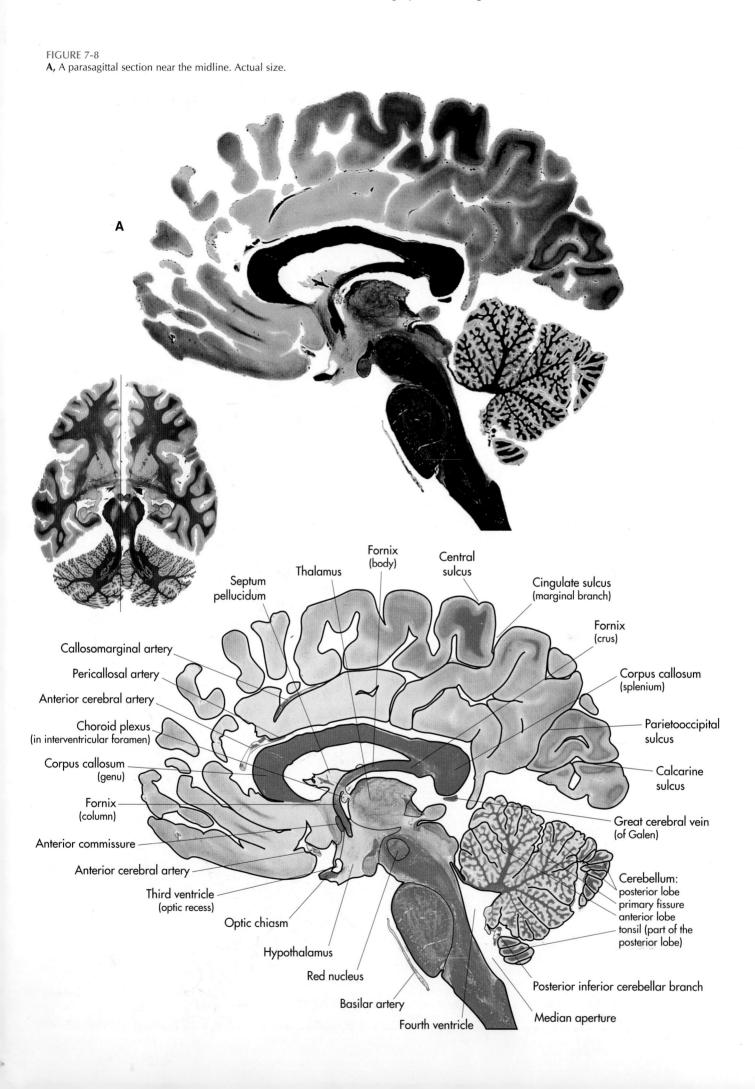

Septum pellucidum

Thalamus

Fornix (body)

Central sulcus

Cingulate sulcus (marginal branch)

Fornix (crus)

Corpus callosum (splenium)

Parietooccipital sulcus

Calcarine sulcus

Great cerebral vein (of Galen)

Cerebellum: posterior lobe primary fissure anterior lobe tonsil (part of the posterior lobe)

Posterior inferior cerebellar branch

Median aperture

Callosomarginal artery

Pericallosal artery

Anterior cerebral artery

Choroid plexus (in interventricular foramen)

Corpus callosum (genu)

Fornix (column)

Anterior commissure

Anterior cerebral artery

Third ventricle (optic recess)

Optic chiasm

Hypothalamus

Red nucleus

Basilar artery

Fourth ventricle

FIGURE 7-8, cont'd.
B, The central region of Figure 7-8, *A,* enlarged to 1.7× actual size.

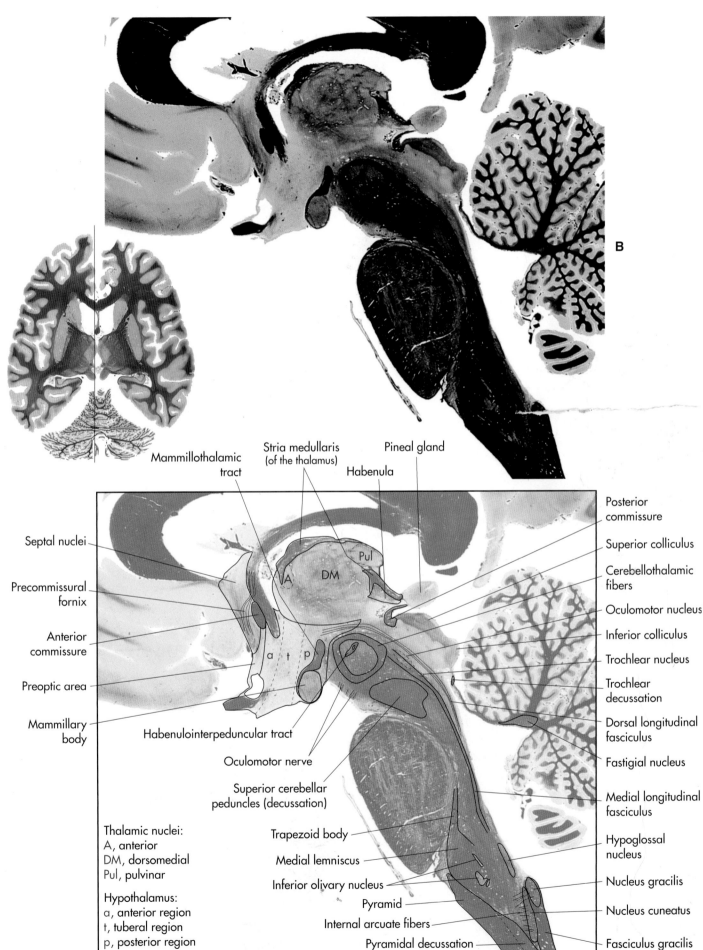

Mammillothalamic tract

Stria medullaris (of the thalamus)

Habenula

Pineal gland

B

Septal nuclei

Precommissural fornix

Anterior commissure

Preoptic area

Mammillary body

Posterior commissure

Superior colliculus

Cerebellothalamic fibers

Oculomotor nucleus

Inferior colliculus

Trochlear nucleus

Trochlear decussation

Dorsal longitudinal fasciculus

Fastigial nucleus

Medial longitudinal fasciculus

Hypoglossal nucleus

Nucleus gracilis

Nucleus cuneatus

Fasciculus gracilis

Pul

A   DM

a   t   p

Habenulointerpeduncular tract

Oculomotor nerve

Superior cerebellar peduncles (decussation)

Trapezoid body

Medial lemniscus

Inferior olivary nucleus

Pyramid

Internal arcuate fibers

Pyramidal decussation

Thalamic nuclei:
A, anterior
DM, dorsomedial
Pul, pulvinar

Hypothalamus:
a, anterior region
t, tuberal region
p, posterior region

FIGURE 7-9
A, A parasagittal section almost exactly in the midline. Actual size.

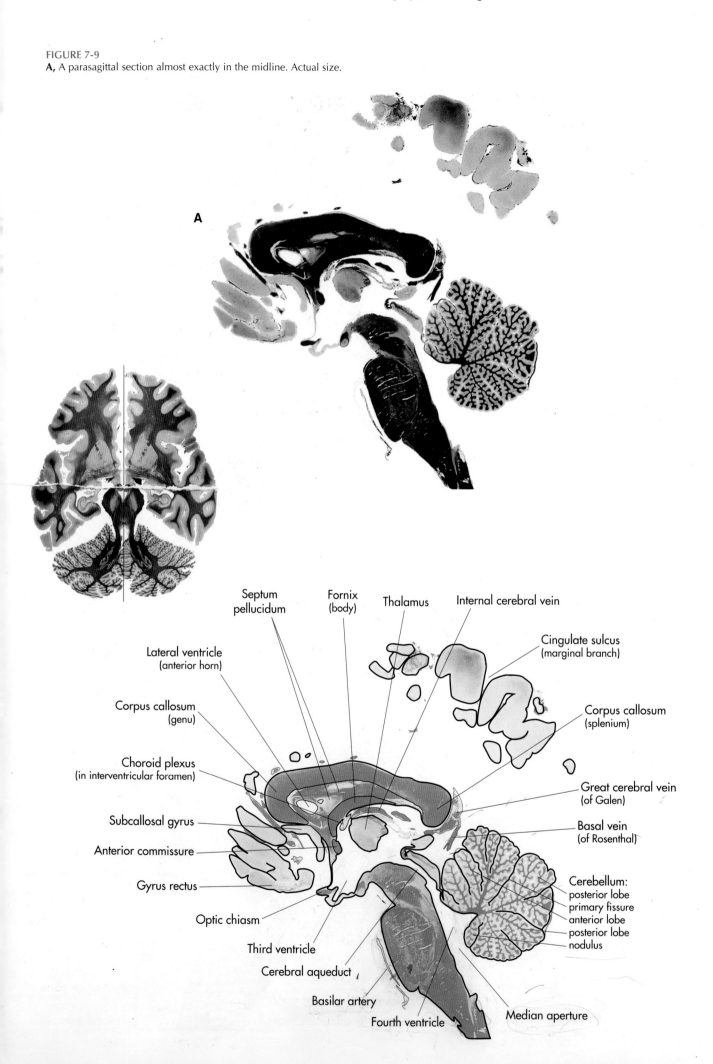

A

Septum
pellucidum

Fornix
(body)

Thalamus

Internal cerebral vein

Lateral ventricle
(anterior horn)

Cingulate sulcus
(marginal branch)

Corpus callosum
(genu)

Corpus callosum
(splenium)

Choroid plexus
(in interventricular foramen)

Great cerebral vein
(of Galen)

Subcallosal gyrus

Basal vein
(of Rosenthal)

Anterior commissure

Cerebellum:
posterior lobe
primary fissure
anterior lobe
posterior lobe
nodulus

Gyrus rectus

Optic chiasm

Third ventricle

Cerebral aqueduct

Basilar artery

Fourth ventricle

Median aperture

FIGURE 7-9, cont'd.
B, The central region of Figure 7-9, *A,* enlarged to 1.7× actual size.

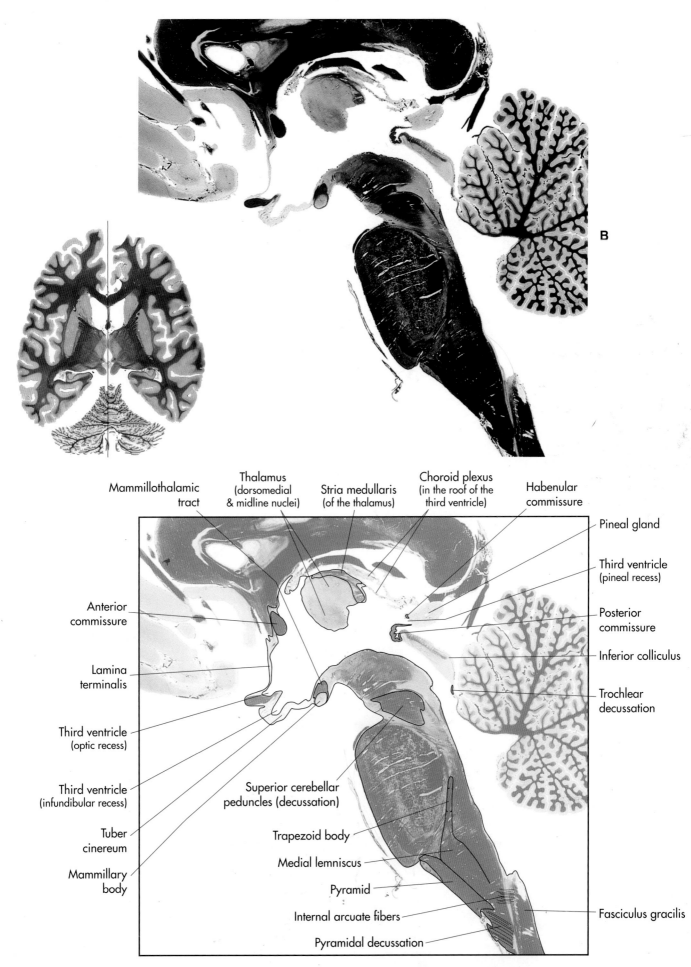

B

Mammillothalamic tract

Thalamus (dorsomedial & midline nuclei)

Stria medullaris (of the thalamus)

Choroid plexus (in the roof of the third ventricle)

Habenular commissure

Pineal gland

Third ventricle (pineal recess)

Anterior commissure

Posterior commissure

Inferior colliculus

Lamina terminalis

Trochlear decussation

Third ventricle (optic recess)

Third ventricle (infundibular recess)

Superior cerebellar peduncles (decussation)

Tuber cinereum

Trapezoid body

Medial lemniscus

Mammillary body

Pyramid

Internal arcuate fibers

Fasciculus gracilis

Pyramidal decussation

chapter 8

FUNCTIONAL SYSTEMS

The preceding chapters presented the major structures seen at individual levels of the central nervous system (CNS) or in particular views of the brain. This chapter is complementary, using many of the same sections and views to indicate the structures and connections involved in particular neurological functions.

We have taken a "bare-bones" approach to this task and indicated only major pathways and connections. Much of the circuitry discussed in standard textbooks was omitted in the interest of simplicity. The locations of neuronal cell bodies, the trajectories of their axons in tracts, and the locations of their synaptic endings are usually indicated by cartoon neurons like this one:

Neuronal cell body ● —— Axon —— ● Synaptic ending

In addition, some anatomical liberties were taken to keep the diagrams relatively simple. The number of lines was minimized by indicating axons as diverging or converging:

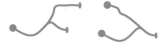

(Axons frequently branch to innervate multiple targets, but this is not what we mean to indicate in any of these figures; moreover, axons from multiple neurons never converge to form a single axon.)

Finally, colors were used to make it easier to follow particular pathways in each figure. Their use is consistent within a given figure, but not across figures: we were unable to devise a meaningful color scheme that would accommodate all the different functional systems. Hence a given color seldom has a functional implication.

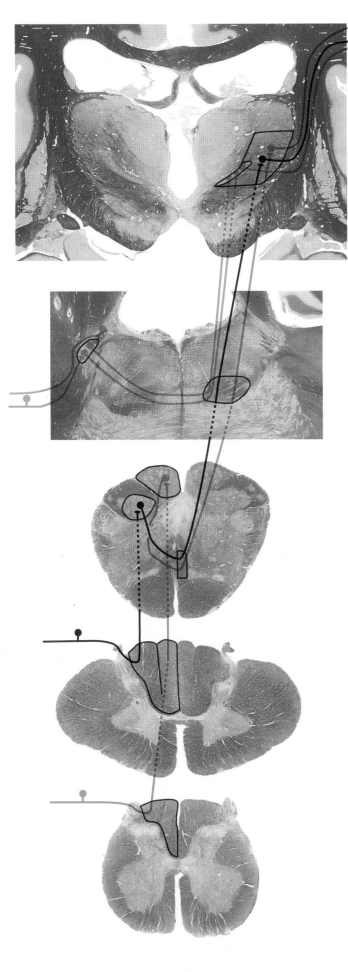

FIGURE 8-1
A, The posterior column–medial lemniscus system.

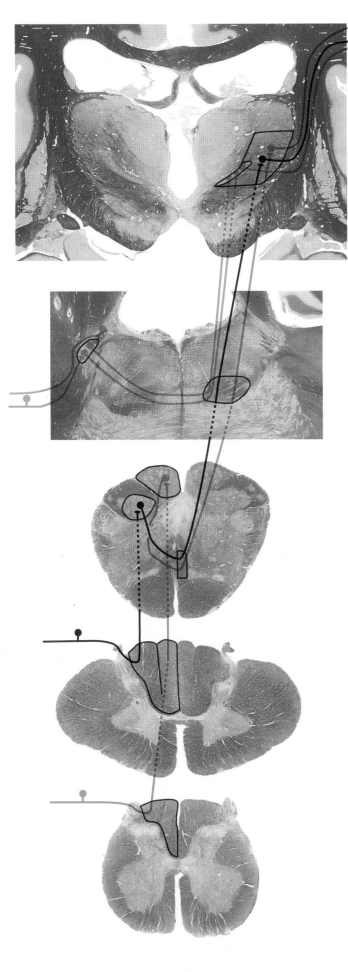

Large-diameter primary afferent fibers, conveying information about limb position and movement and the details of tactile stimuli, enter the spinal cord in the medial division of each dorsal root. The principal route through which this information reaches consciousness is the posterior column–medial lemniscus pathway. Branches of the primary afferents ascend through the ipsilateral posterior funiculus. Entering fibers add onto the lateral aspect of fibers already present in the posterior funiculus (see Figure 8-1, *B [inset]*), so by the time they reach the medulla fibers conveying information from the leg are located in the more medial fasciculus gracilis and those conveying information from the arm in the more lateral fasciculus cuneatus. This is the beginning of a somatotopic arrangement that is maintained (with some twists and turns) throughout the remainder of this pathway.

Each posterior column terminates in the ipsilateral posterior column nuclei (nuclei gracilis and cuneatus), whose axons cross the midline and ascend to the ventral posterolateral (VPL) nucleus of the thalamus. VPL in turn projects to primary somatosensory cortex in the postcentral gyrus.

An analogous pathway conveying similar information from the face involves primary afferents with cell bodies in the trigeminal ganglion and the mesencephalic nucleus of the trigeminal nerve (see Figure 8-4). Central processes of these afferents terminate in the main sensory nucleus of the trigeminal nerve. Their axons cross the midline, join the somatotopically appropriate region of the medial lemniscus, and ascend to the ventral posteromedial (VPM) nucleus of the thalamus. VPM in turn projects to the face area of the postcentral gyrus.

Tactile and proprioceptive information can also reach consciousness by way of postsynaptic fibers arising from spinal cord neurons. Some of these projections travel in the posterior columns, but others travel in pathways outside the posterior funiculus (e.g., tactile information in the anterolateral system described in Figure 8-2), so posterior column damage does not cause total loss of touch and position sensation.

FIGURE 8-1, cont'd.
B, The posterior column–medial lemniscus system, continued. *(Inset re-drawn from Mettler FA: Neuroanatomy, ed 2, St. Louis, 1948, Mosby.)*

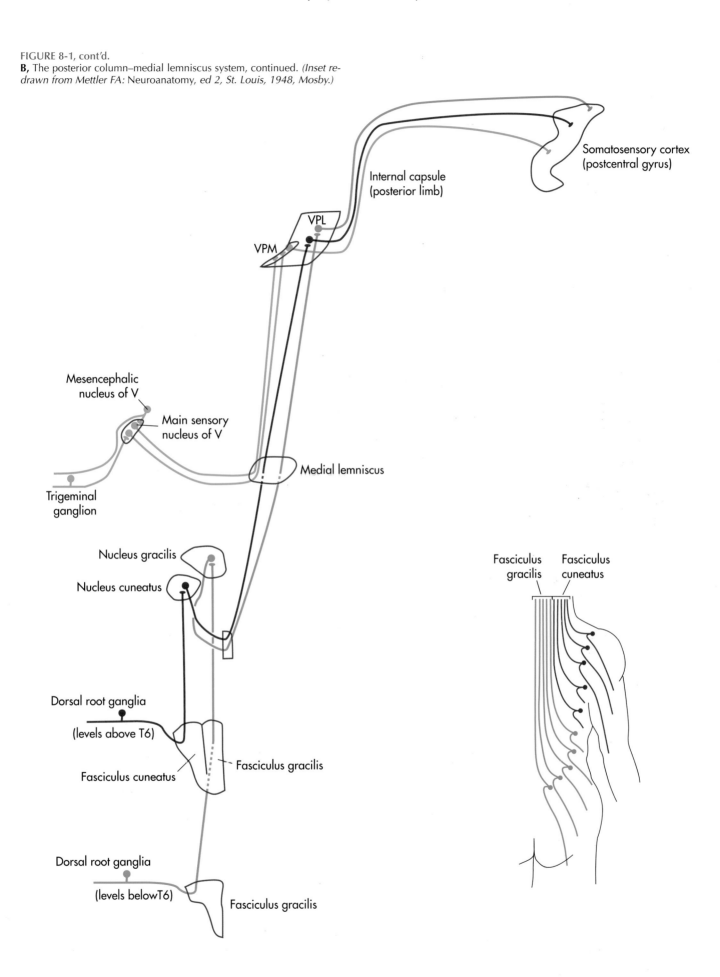

FIGURE 8-2
A, The anterolateral system.

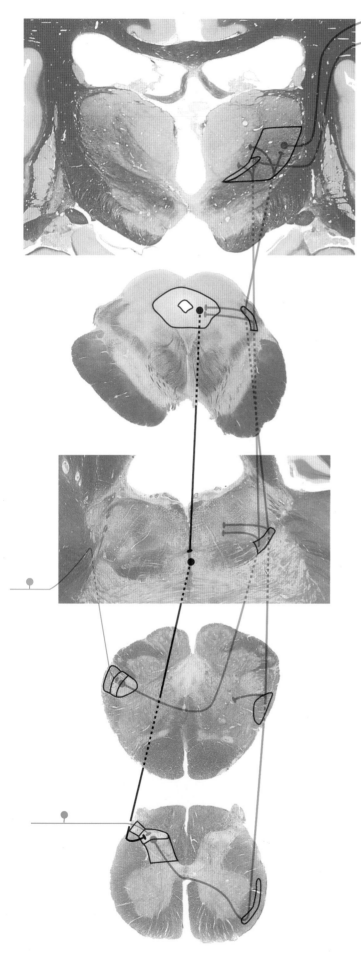

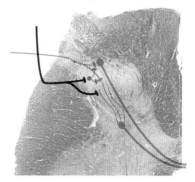

Small-diameter afferent fibers conveying pain and temperature (and a limited amount of tactile) information enter the spinal cord in the lateral division of each dorsal root. The principal route through which this information reaches consciousness is the spinothalamic tract. Primary afferents terminate on tract cells in the posterior horn, whose axons cross and join the spinothalamic tract, adding onto the ventromedial aspect of fibers already present. This initiates a somatotopic arrangement that is maintained (relatively unchanged) throughout the pathway. Spinothalamic fibers then ascend to VPL of the thalamus, which projects to primary somatosensory cortex in the postcentral gyrus.

The analogous trigeminal pathway involves trigeminal ganglion cells whose central processes descend through the spinal trigeminal tract to caudal parts of the spinal trigeminal nucleus (see Figure 8-4). Axons of these second-order neurons cross the midline, join the somatotopically appropriate region of the spinothalamic tract, and ascend to VPM of the thalamus. VPM in turn projects to the face area of the postcentral gyrus.

Pain (and presumably temperature) information is in fact more widely distributed than this simplified account would indicate and reaches the reticular formation, additional thalamic nuclei, and multiple cortical areas. Several additional pain pathways travel with or near the spinothalamic tract and all are commonly referred to collectively as the *anterolateral system.*

Access to the spinothalamic tract is modulated by small neurons of the substantia gelatinosa (and at several other sites). One important pain-control pathway originates in the periaqueductal gray matter of the midbrain and involves a relay in the raphe nuclei (see Figure 8-34) and nearby reticular formation of the medulla and caudal pons.

FIGURE 8-2, cont'd.
B, The anterolateral system, continued.

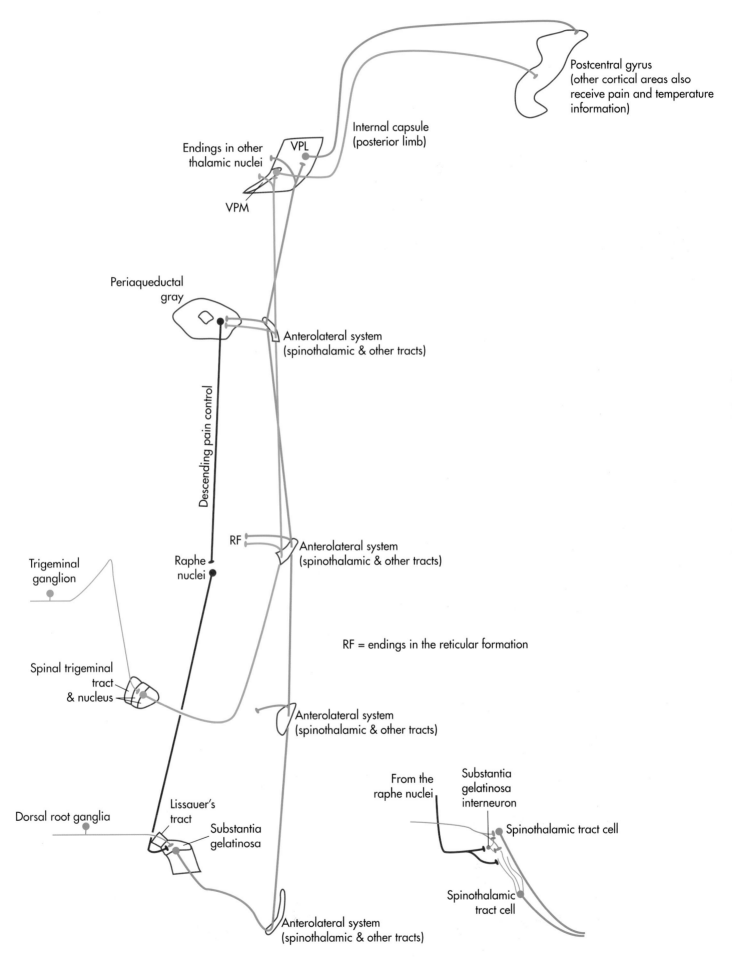

FIGURE 8-3
A, The corticospinal tract.

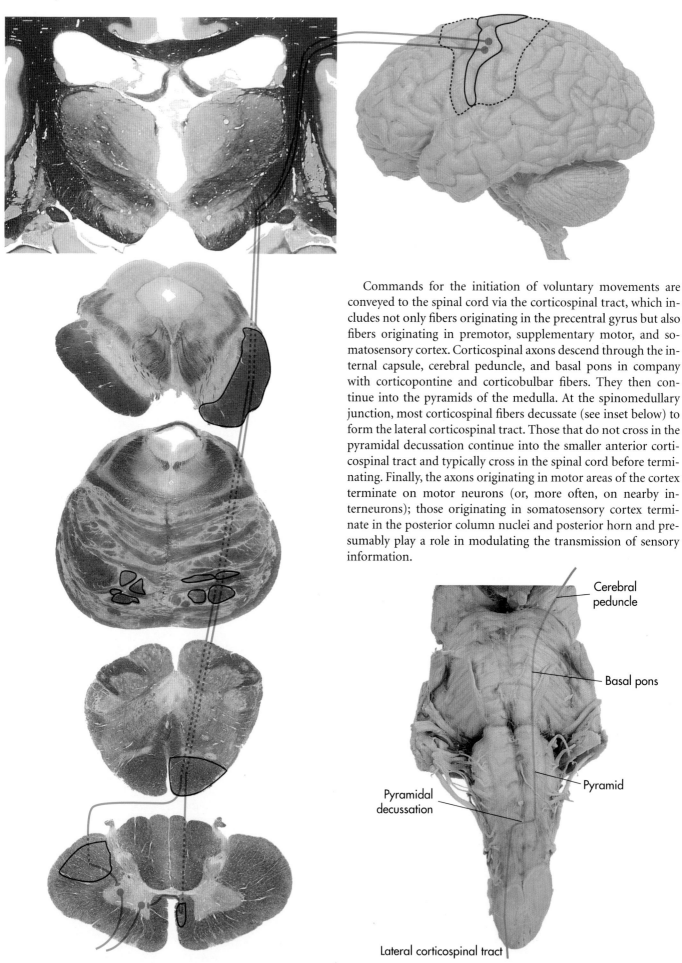

Commands for the initiation of voluntary movements are conveyed to the spinal cord via the corticospinal tract, which includes not only fibers originating in the precentral gyrus but also fibers originating in premotor, supplementary motor, and somatosensory cortex. Corticospinal axons descend through the internal capsule, cerebral peduncle, and basal pons in company with corticopontine and corticobulbar fibers. They then continue into the pyramids of the medulla. At the spinomedullary junction, most corticospinal fibers decussate (see inset below) to form the lateral corticospinal tract. Those that do not cross in the pyramidal decussation continue into the smaller anterior corticospinal tract and typically cross in the spinal cord before terminating. Finally, the axons originating in motor areas of the cortex terminate on motor neurons (or, more often, on nearby interneurons); those originating in somatosensory cortex terminate in the posterior column nuclei and posterior horn and presumably play a role in modulating the transmission of sensory information.

Cerebral peduncle

Basal pons

Pyramid

Pyramidal decussation

Lateral corticospinal tract

FIGURE 8-3, cont'd.
B, The corticospinal tract, continued.

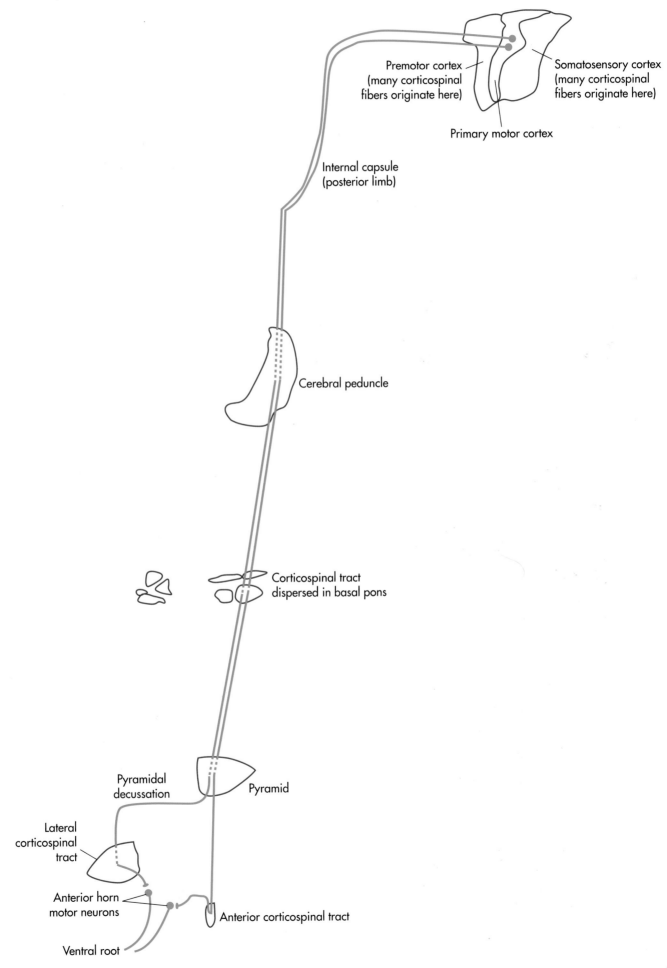

Premotor cortex
(many corticospinal
fibers originate here)

Somatosensory cortex
(many corticospinal
fibers originate here)

Primary motor cortex

Internal capsule
(posterior limb)

Cerebral peduncle

Corticospinal tract
dispersed in basal pons

Pyramidal
decussation

Pyramid

Lateral
corticospinal
tract

Anterior horn
motor neurons

Anterior corticospinal tract

Ventral root

FIGURE 8-4
A, Central connections of the trigeminal nerve.

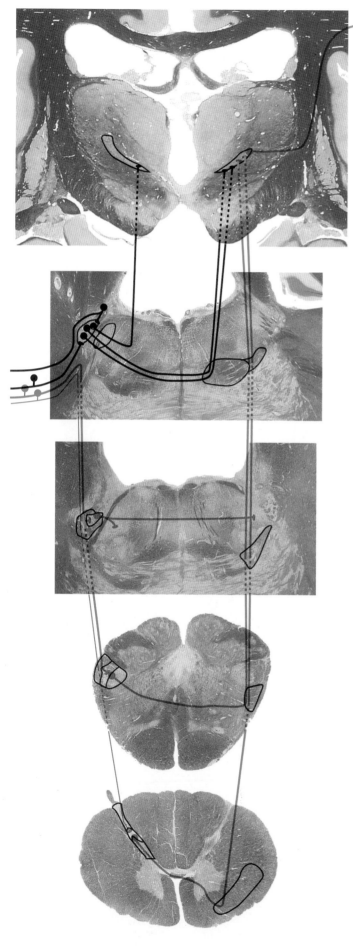
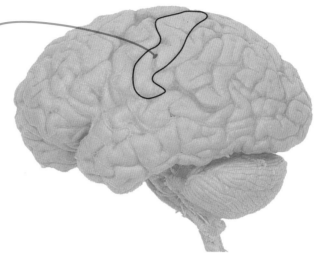

The trigeminal nerve conveys somatic sensory information from most of the head, and it is also the motor nerve for most muscles of mastication. Connections of the trigeminal motor nucleus are noted in Figure 8-11, and sensory connections are reviewed here. The connections of somatosensory components bear many similarities to those of spinal nerves (see Figures 8-1 and 8-2), but there are important differences as well.

Large-diameter trigeminal afferents have cell bodies in the trigeminal ganglion or in the mesencephalic nucleus of the trigeminal (in effect, a bit of the trigeminal ganglion located within the CNS instead of in the periphery). Many central processes terminate in the main sensory nucleus of the trigeminal, which in turn projects through the contralateral medial lemniscus to the VPM of the thalamus. (Part of the main sensory nucleus, where the mouth is represented, sends an uncrossed projection, the dorsal trigeminal tract, to the ipsilateral VPM; the functional significance of this uncrossed projection is unclear.) Other central processes project to the trigeminal motor nucleus as part of the masseter stretch reflex arc, or to trigeminocerebellar neurons in rostral parts of the spinal trigeminal nucleus.

Small-diameter trigeminal afferents, all with cell bodies in the trigeminal ganglion, travel through the spinal trigeminal tract to termination sites at various levels of the spinal trigeminal nucleus. (The spinal trigeminal tract and nucleus merge smoothly with Lissauer's tract and the posterior horn, respectively, of the upper cervical spinal cord.) The most caudal levels of the spinal trigeminal nucleus convey information about facial pain and temperature to VPM. More rostral levels participate in trigeminocerebellar projections and in other reflexes, notably the bilateral blink reflex in response to an object touching either cornea.

FIGURE 8-4, cont'd.
B, Central connections of the trigeminal nerve, continued.

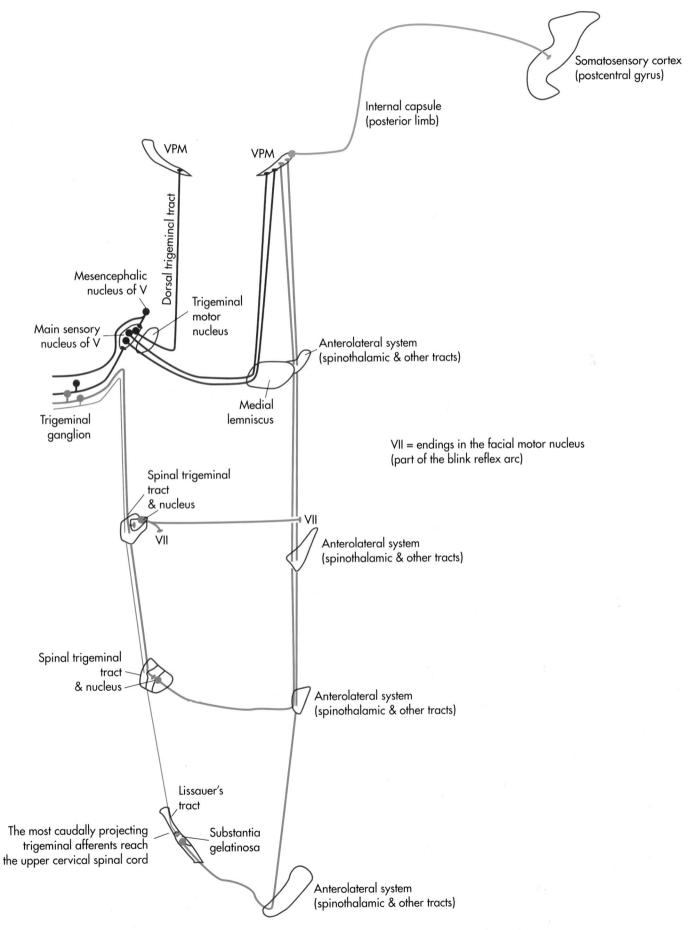

FIGURE 8-5
A, Central gustatory connections.

What we commonly refer to as "taste" is actually a complex sensation. Sensory information from taste buds is an important contributor, but this is combined with information from olfactory receptors (aroma) and trigeminal endings (texture, spiciness, temperature). To avoid ambiguity, the sensations initiated in taste buds are referred to as *gustatory* sensations.

The receptor cells in taste buds synapse on peripheral processes of fibers in the facial (VII), glossopharyngeal (IX), and vagus (X) nerves. Facial endings innervate taste buds on the anterior two thirds of the tongue, glossopharyngeal endings innervate those on the posterior third, and vagal endings innervate scattered taste buds of the epiglottis and esophagus. Central processes of these gustatory primary afferents travel through the solitary tract to reach second-order neurons in the nucleus of the solitary tract.

Second-order gustatory neurons influence feeding-related behavior and autonomic functions by projecting to the dorsal motor nucleus of the vagus, to the nearby reticular formation, and even to preganglionic sympathetic neurons in the spinal cord (not indicated in the accompanying figures). Conscious perception of taste is mediated by an uncrossed projection from the nucleus of the solitary tract to the thalamus (VPM), and from there to gustatory cortex in the insula and adjacent frontal operculum.

Gustatory information also reaches the hypothalamus and amygdala, where it influences metabolic regulation and feelings of hunger, satiety, and pleasantness or unpleasantness accompanying various tastes. The route utilized involves, at least partially, a projection from gustatory cortex to the amygdala. In many animals, gustatory information is also transmitted to the hypothalamus and amygdala more directly, through a projection from the parabrachial nucleus of the pontine reticular formation. Whether this pathway is important in humans is uncertain, as implied by question marks in Figure 8-5, *B.*

FIGURE 8-5, cont'd.
B, Central gustatory connections, continued. *(Tongue inset modified from Nolte J:* The human brain, *ed 4, St. Louis, 1999, Mosby.)*

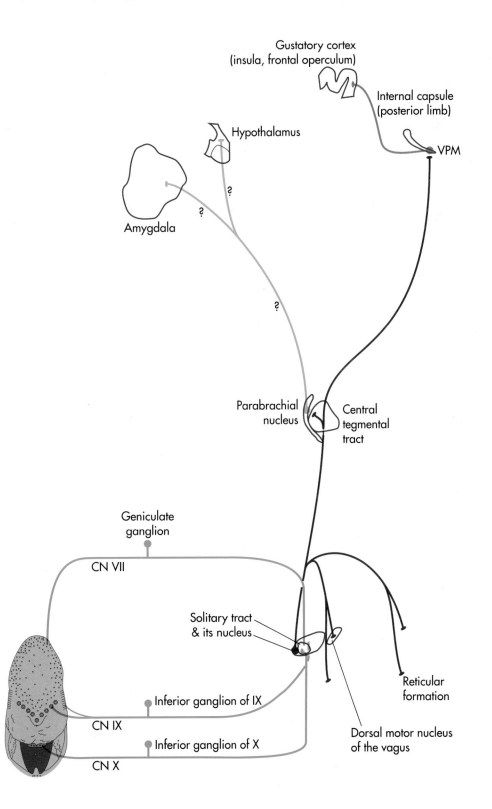

FIGURE 8-6
A, Central olfactory connections. *(Prosection from Nolte J:* The human brain, *ed 4, St. Louis, 1999, Mosby.)*

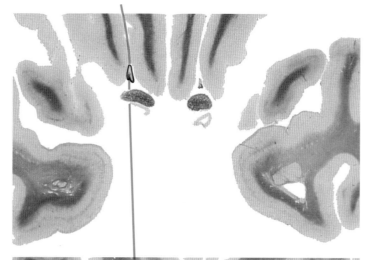

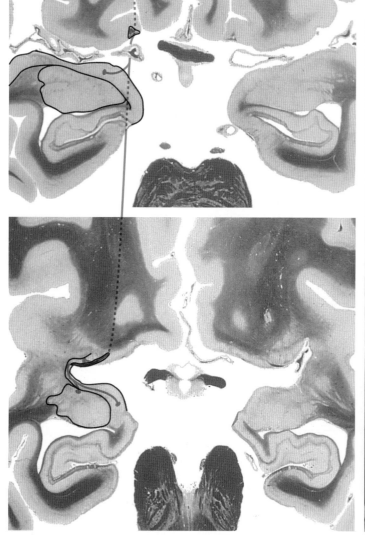

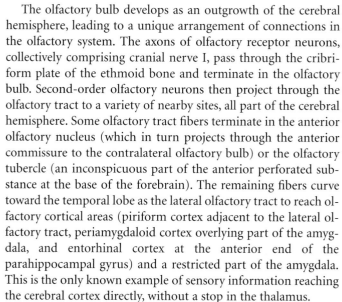

The olfactory bulb develops as an outgrowth of the cerebral hemisphere, leading to a unique arrangement of connections in the olfactory system. The axons of olfactory receptor neurons, collectively comprising cranial nerve I, pass through the cribriform plate of the ethmoid bone and terminate in the olfactory bulb. Second-order olfactory neurons then project through the olfactory tract to a variety of nearby sites, all part of the cerebral hemisphere. Some olfactory tract fibers terminate in the anterior olfactory nucleus (which in turn projects through the anterior commissure to the contralateral olfactory bulb) or the olfactory tubercle (an inconspicuous part of the anterior perforated substance at the base of the forebrain). The remaining fibers curve toward the temporal lobe as the lateral olfactory tract to reach olfactory cortical areas (piriform cortex adjacent to the lateral olfactory tract, periamygdaloid cortex overlying part of the amygdala, and entorhinal cortex at the anterior end of the parahippocampal gyrus) and a restricted part of the amygdala. This is the only known example of sensory information reaching the cerebral cortex directly, without a stop in the thalamus.

Olfactory information is subsequently distributed more widely, both by projections from these primary olfactory receiving areas and by relays in the thalamus.

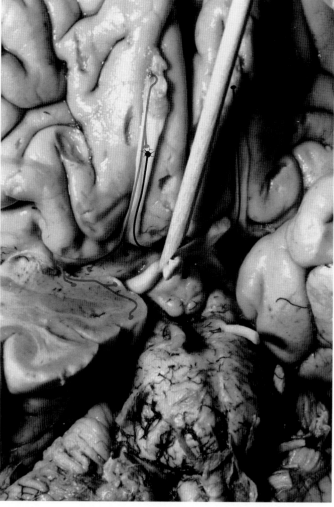

FIGURE 8-6, cont'd.
B, Central olfactory connections, continued.

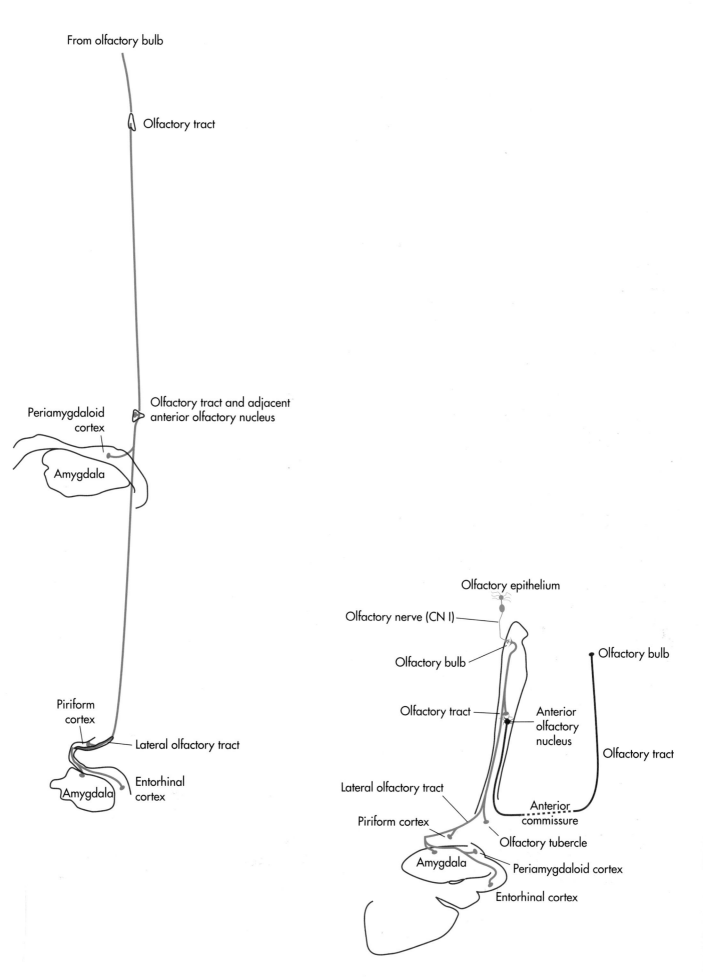

FIGURE 8-7
A, The auditory system.

Auditory information reaches the brainstem via the cochlear division of cranial nerve VIII, a collection of primary afferent fibers with cell bodies in the spiral ganglion, peripheral processes that innervate cochlear hair cells, and central processes that terminate in the dorsal and ventral cochlear nuclei at the pontomedullary junction.

In contrast to some other sensory systems, the second-order neurons of the cochlear nuclei project bilaterally (crossing in the trapezoid body) to higher levels of the auditory system, allowing for sound localization by comparing inputs from the two ears. The first site where such binaural comparisons occur is the superior olivary nucleus. Efferents from each superior olivary nucleus, together with crossed and uncrossed projections from the cochlear nuclei, ascend to the inferior colliculus through the lateral lemniscus. The inferior colliculus then projects through the brachium of the inferior colliculus to the medial geniculate nucleus of the thalamus, which in turn projects to auditory cortex in the temporal lobe. Primary auditory cortex is located in the aptly named transverse temporal gyri (of Heschl) on the superior surface of the superior temporal gyrus.

Because beyond the cochlear nuclei both ears are represented in the auditory pathway on each side of the CNS, serious hearing loss restricted to one ear implies damage at the level of the cochlear nuclei or (more likely) the middle or inner ear.

FIGURE 8-7, cont'd.
B, The auditory system, continued. *(Prosection from Nolte J: The human brain, ed 4, St. Louis, 1999, Mosby.)*

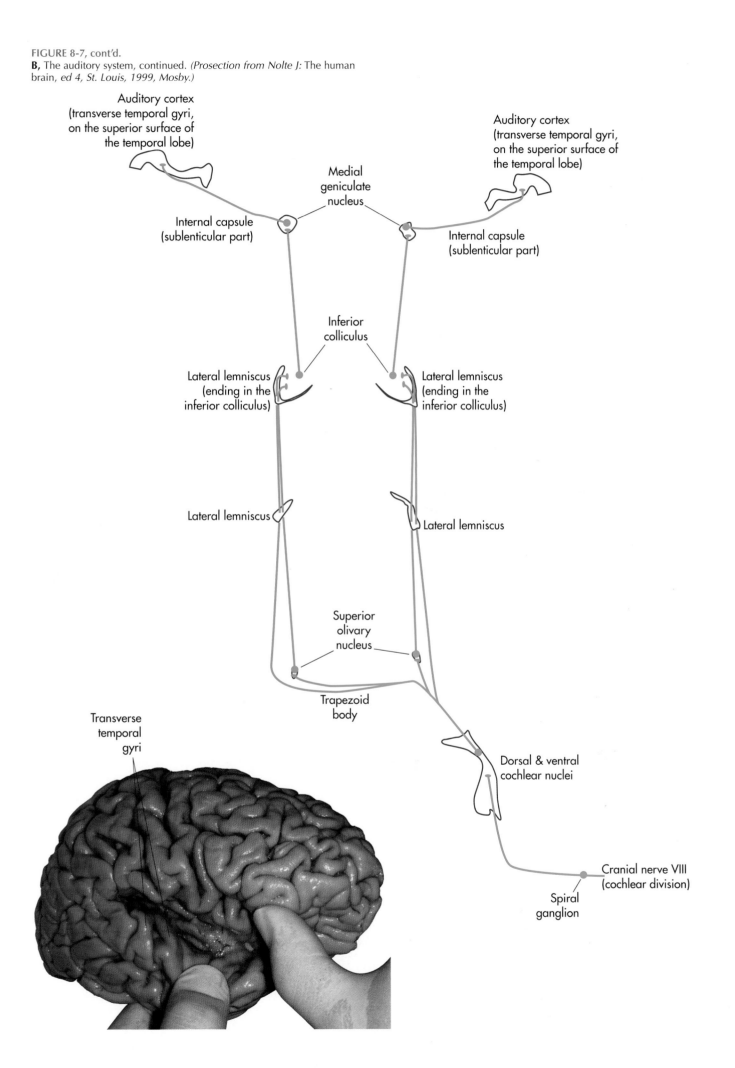

Auditory cortex
(transverse temporal gyri,
on the superior surface of
the temporal lobe)

Auditory cortex
(transverse temporal gyri,
on the superior surface of
the temporal lobe)

Medial
geniculate
nucleus

Internal capsule
(sublenticular part)

Internal capsule
(sublenticular part)

Inferior
colliculus

Lateral lemniscus
(ending in the
inferior colliculus)

Lateral lemniscus
(ending in the
inferior colliculus)

Lateral lemniscus

Lateral lemniscus

Superior
olivary
nucleus

Trapezoid
body

Transverse
temporal
gyri

Dorsal & ventral
cochlear nuclei

Cranial nerve VIII
(cochlear division)

Spiral
ganglion

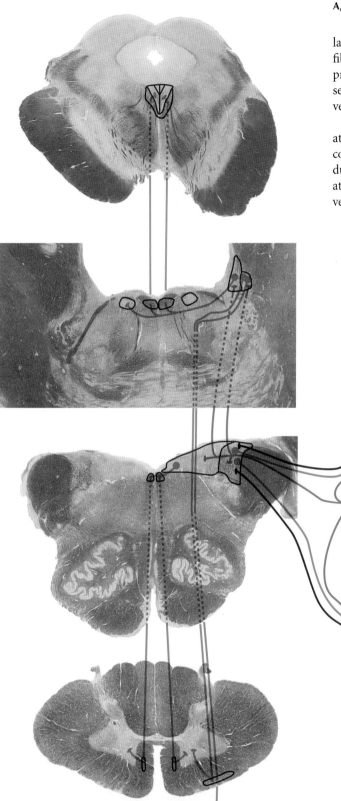

FIGURE 8-8
A, The vestibular system.

Vestibular information reaches the brainstem via the vestibular division of cranial nerve VIII, a collection of primary afferent fibers with cell bodies in the vestibular ganglion, peripheral processes that innervate hair cells in the utricle, saccule, and semicircular canals, and central processes that terminate in the vestibular nuclei of the rostral medulla and caudal pons.

The vestibular nuclei then project to the spinal cord (to mediate postural responses to linear and angular acceleration, and to coordinate head movements with eye movements) and to the abducens, trochlear (not shown), and oculomotor nuclei (to mediate eye movements compensating for head movements—the vestibuloocular reflex).

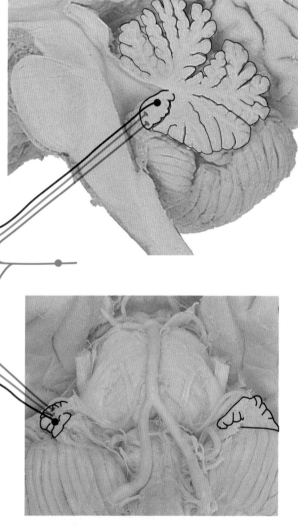

Abundant interconnections between the vestibular nuclei and the cerebellum (particularly the flocculonodular lobe and parts of the vermis) assist in these tasks. Finally, there is a projection (not shown) from the vestibular nuclei to the thalamus through which changes in head position or motion reach consciousness.

The lateral and medial vestibulospinal tracts arise primarily from the lateral and medial vestibular nuclei, respectively. Other vestibular connections, however, are shared among all the nuclei; the apparently exclusive connections in Figure 8-8, *B* are merely a mechanism for minimizing the number of lines in the figure.

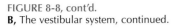

FIGURE 8-8, cont'd.
B, The vestibular system, continued.

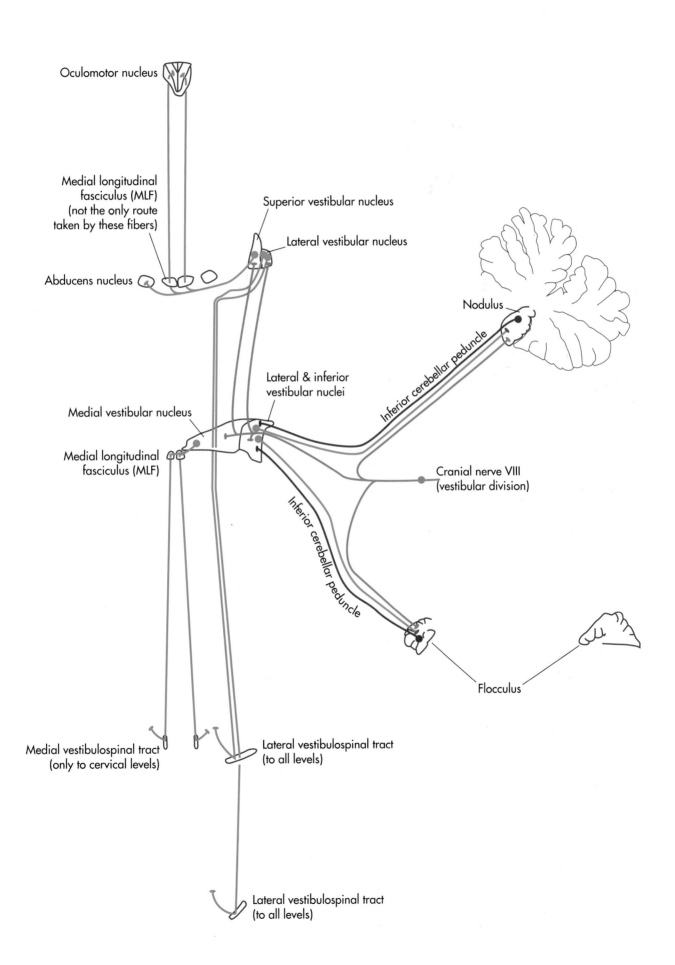

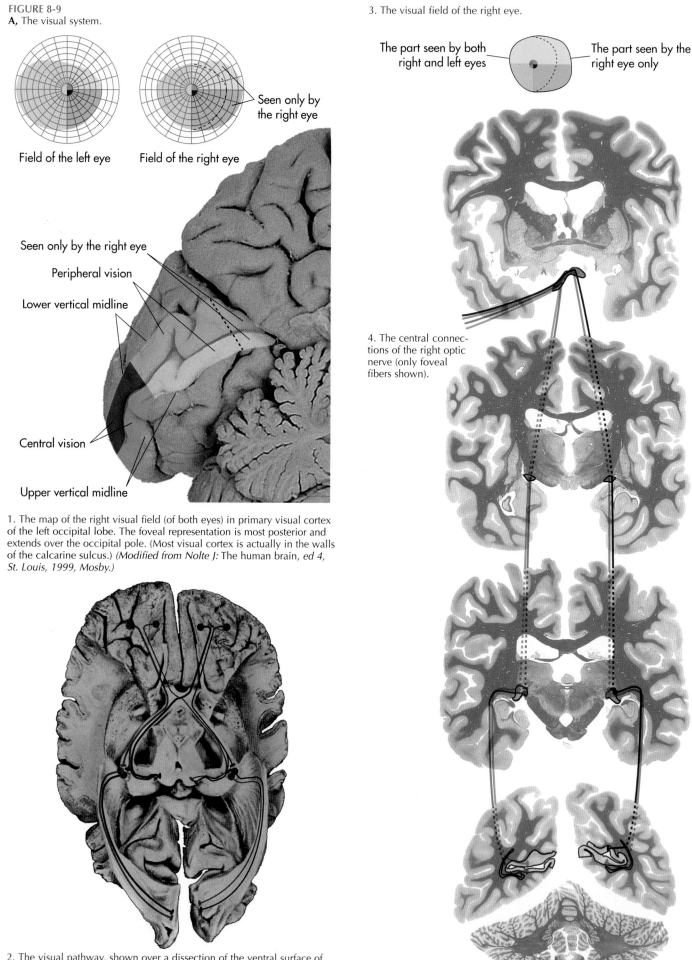

FIGURE 8-9
A, The visual system.

Field of the left eye   Field of the right eye

Seen only by the right eye

Seen only by the right eye
Peripheral vision
Lower vertical midline

Central vision

Upper vertical midline

1. The map of the right visual field (of both eyes) in primary visual cortex of the left occipital lobe. The foveal representation is most posterior and extends over the occipital pole. (Most visual cortex is actually in the walls of the calcarine sulcus.) *(Modified from Nolte J: The human brain, ed 4, St. Louis, 1999, Mosby.)*

2. The visual pathway, shown over a dissection of the ventral surface of the brain. *(Modified from Ludwig E, Klingler J: Atlas cerebri humani, Boston, 1956, Little, Brown & Co.)*

3. The visual field of the right eye.

The part seen by both right and left eyes   The part seen by the right eye only

4. The central connections of the right optic nerve (only foveal fibers shown).

FIGURE 8-9, cont'd.
B, The visual system, continued.

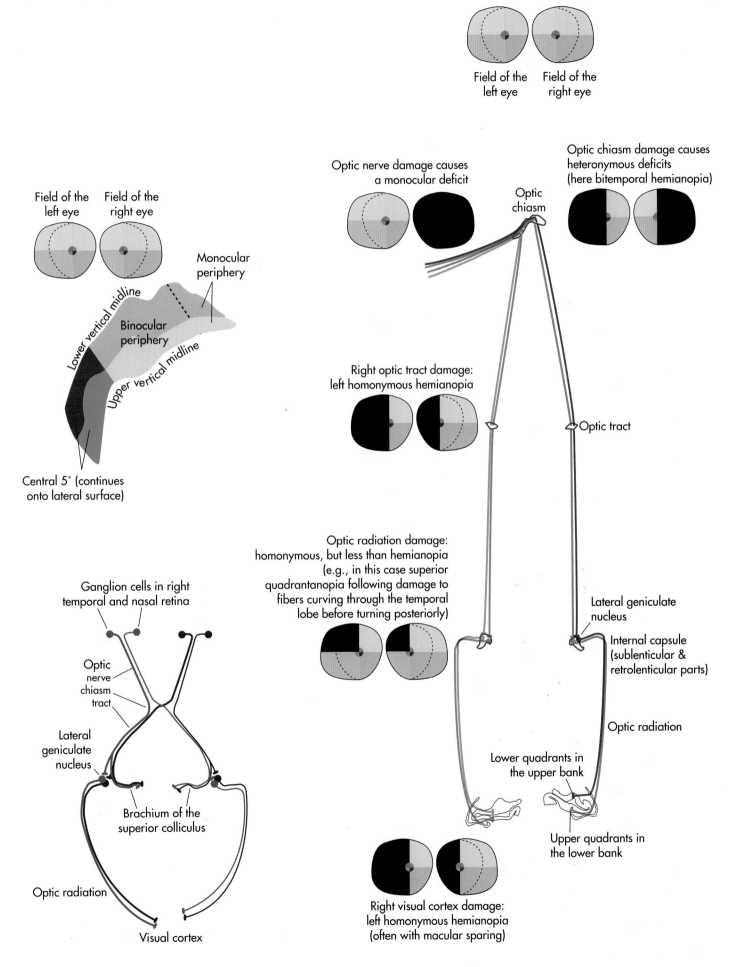

FIGURE 8-10
Cranial nerve nuclei that innervate ordinary skeletal muscle.

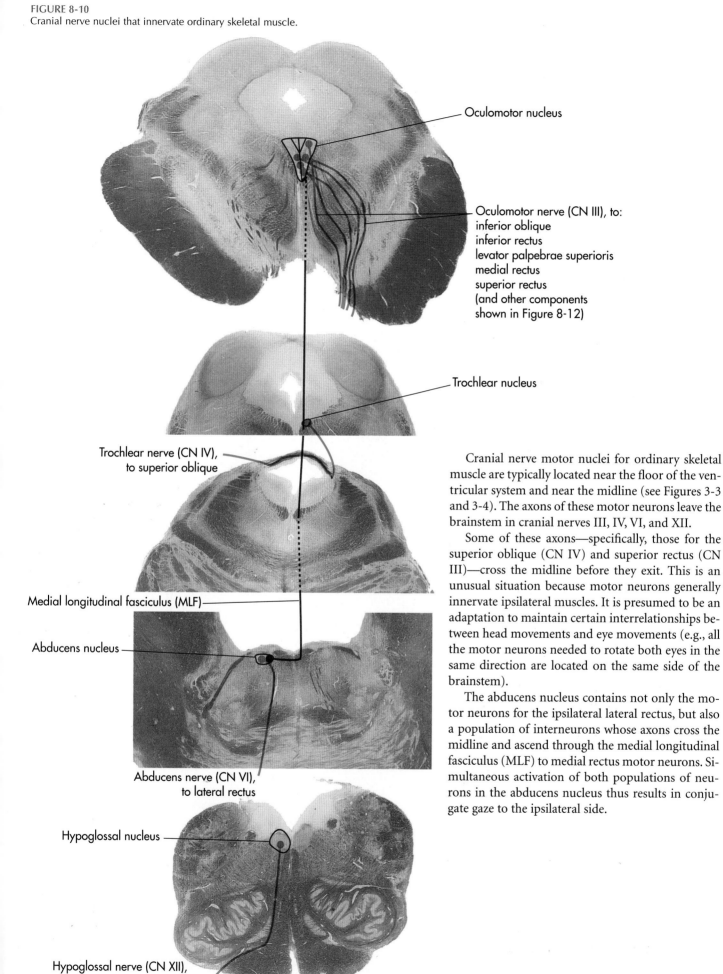

Oculomotor nucleus

Oculomotor nerve (CN III), to:
inferior oblique
inferior rectus
levator palpebrae superioris
medial rectus
superior rectus
(and other components
shown in Figure 8-12)

Trochlear nucleus

Trochlear nerve (CN IV),
to superior oblique

Medial longitudinal fasciculus (MLF)

Abducens nucleus

Abducens nerve (CN VI),
to lateral rectus

Hypoglossal nucleus

Hypoglossal nerve (CN XII),
to tongue muscles

Cranial nerve motor nuclei for ordinary skeletal muscle are typically located near the floor of the ventricular system and near the midline (see Figures 3-3 and 3-4). The axons of these motor neurons leave the brainstem in cranial nerves III, IV, VI, and XII.

Some of these axons—specifically, those for the superior oblique (CN IV) and superior rectus (CN III)—cross the midline before they exit. This is an unusual situation because motor neurons generally innervate ipsilateral muscles. It is presumed to be an adaptation to maintain certain interrelationships between head movements and eye movements (e.g., all the motor neurons needed to rotate both eyes in the same direction are located on the same side of the brainstem).

The abducens nucleus contains not only the motor neurons for the ipsilateral lateral rectus, but also a population of interneurons whose axons cross the midline and ascend through the medial longitudinal fasciculus (MLF) to medial rectus motor neurons. Simultaneous activation of both populations of neurons in the abducens nucleus thus results in conjugate gaze to the ipsilateral side.

FIGURE 8-11
Cranial nerve nuclei that innervate skeletal muscle of branchial arch origin.

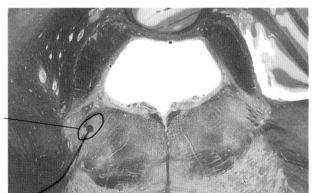

Trigeminal motor nucleus

Trigeminal nerve (CN V, motor root), to:
Muscles of mastication (masseter,
temporalis, pterygoids, others);
tensor tympani

Internal genu
of the facial nerve

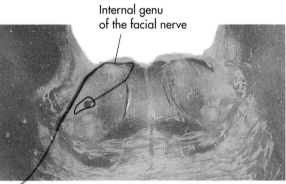

Facial nerve (CN VII), to:
buccinator, orbicularis oris,
orbicularis oculi, other facial muscles;
stapedius
(see Figure 8-12 for other components)

Cranial nerve motor nuclei for skeletal muscle derived embryologically from branchial arches are typically located farther from both the midline and the floor of the ventricular system than are their counterparts for ordinary skeletal muscle (see Figures 3-3 and 3-4).

The axons of these motor neurons leave the brainstem in cranial nerves V, VII, IX, X, and XI. Many of them make an odd, hairpin turn before their exit. Axons leaving the facial motor nucleus provide the most striking example, hooking around the abducens nucleus in an internal genu (accounting for the facial colliculus in the floor of the fourth ventricle—see Figure 1-8, *A*).

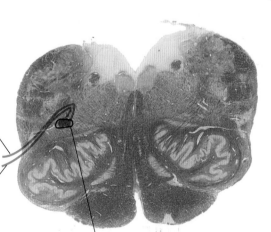

Glossopharyngeal nerve (CN IX),
to stylopharyngeus
(see Figure 8-12 for other components)

Vagus nerve (CN X),
to laryngeal and pharyngeal muscles
(see Figure 8-12 for other components)

Nucleus ambiguus (extends longitudinally
through the rostral medulla)

Accessory nerve (CN XI), to:
sternocleidomastoid
trapezius

Accessory nucleus
(extends longitudinally from the
caudal medulla through C5)

FIGURE 8-12
A, Visceral and gustatory afferents (right side of the figure); preganglionic sympathetic and parasympathetic neurons (left side of the figure). Relatively minor elements (e.g., visceral afferents in the facial nerve) and some elements lacking a distinct CNS nucleus (e.g., preganglionic parasympathetics mediating lacrimation and salivation via the facial and glossopharyngeal nerves) were omitted.

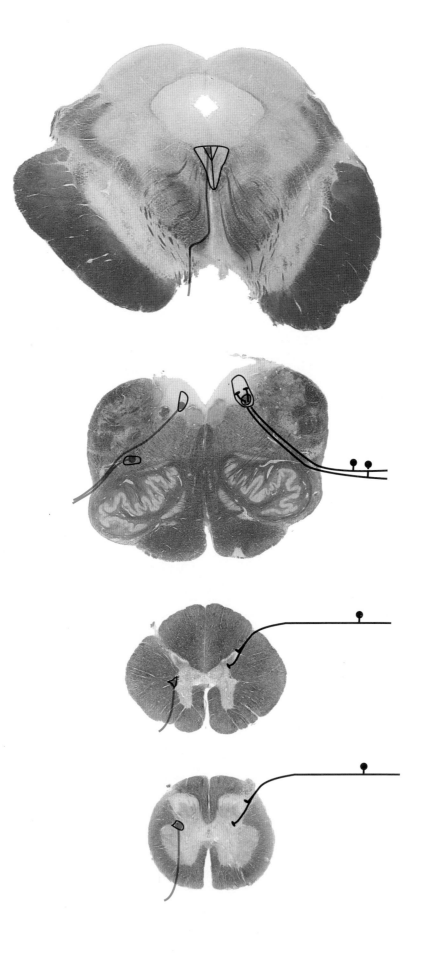

FIGURE 8-12
B, Visceral afferents and efferents, continued.

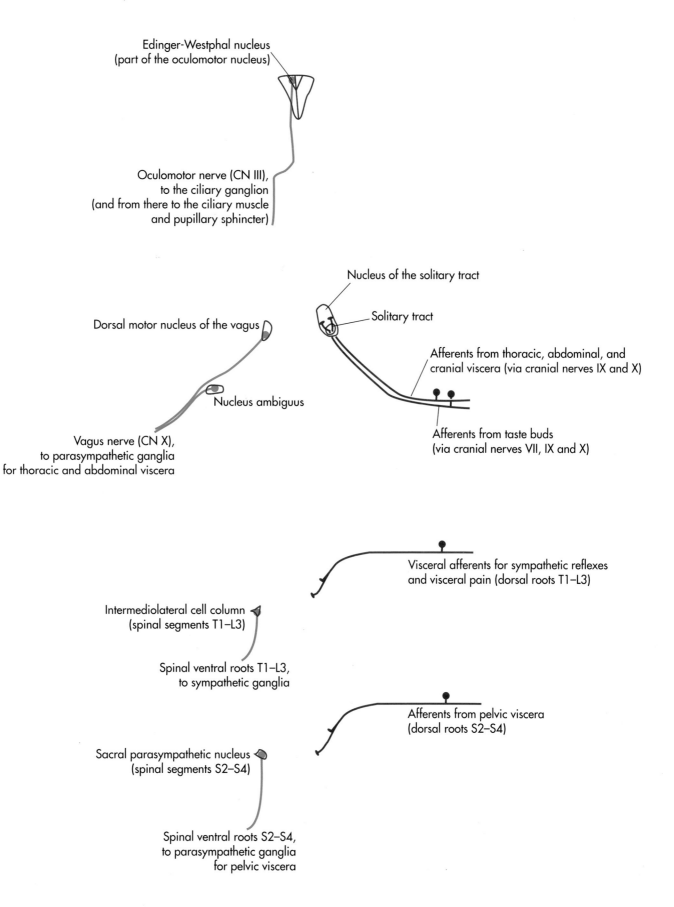

Edinger-Westphal nucleus
(part of the oculomotor nucleus)

Oculomotor nerve (CN III),
to the ciliary ganglion
(and from there to the ciliary muscle
and pupillary sphincter)

Nucleus of the solitary tract

Solitary tract

Dorsal motor nucleus of the vagus

Afferents from thoracic, abdominal, and
cranial viscera (via cranial nerves IX and X)

Nucleus ambiguus

Afferents from taste buds
(via cranial nerves VII, IX and X)

Vagus nerve (CN X),
to parasympathetic ganglia
for thoracic and abdominal viscera

Visceral afferents for sympathetic reflexes
and visceral pain (dorsal roots T1–L3)

Intermediolateral cell column
(spinal segments T1–L3)

Spinal ventral roots T1–L3,
to sympathetic ganglia

Afferents from pelvic viscera
(dorsal roots S2–S4)

Sacral parasympathetic nucleus
(spinal segments S2–S4)

Spinal ventral roots S2–S4,
to parasympathetic ganglia
for pelvic viscera

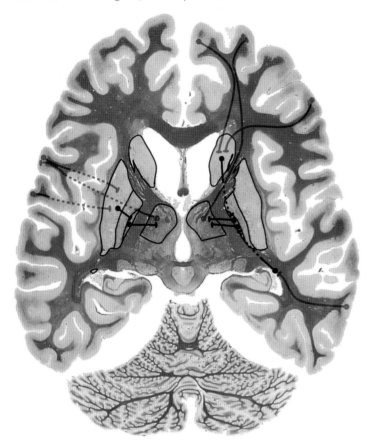

The basal ganglia, which include the striatum,* globus pallidus, subthalamic nucleus, and substantia nigra, are prominently involved in motor control (and in cognitive functions as well, in ways less well understood). They affect movement not by projecting to motor neurons in the spinal cord or brainstem, but rather by influencing the output of the cerebral cortex. The principal anatomical circuit underlying this influence is a series of parallel loops of the type indicated in the inset below: a relatively widespread area of cerebral cortex projects to a particular region of the striatum, which by way of the globus pallidus and thalamus feeds back to the cerebral cortex (typically to a frontal or limbic area).

Most parts of the cerebral cortex, and the hippocampus and amygdala as well, participate in such loops. Association areas of cortex are related most prominently to the caudate nucleus, somatosensory and motor cortex to the putamen, and limbic areas to the ventral striatum.

The subthalamic nucleus and substantia nigra form parts of additional basal ganglia circuitry, as indicated in Figures 8-16 and 8-17.

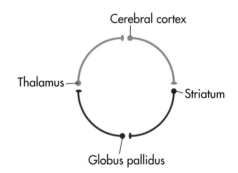

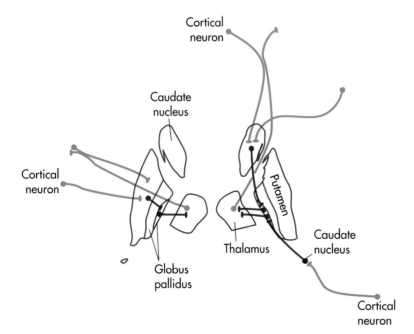

Striatum refers to the combination of caudate nucleus, putamen, and ventral striatum (itself a combination of nucleus accumbens and adjacent parts of the caudate, putamen, and basal forebrain).

FIGURE 8-14
Connections of the striatum; afferents on the left, efferents on the right. Excitatory connections are shown in green, inhibitory connections in red. (Inputs from the compact part of the substantia nigra are shown in a third color because they excite some striatal neurons and inhibit others.)

The most prominent afferents to the striatum arise in the cerebral cortex, substantia nigra (compact part), and intralaminar nuclei of the thalamus (especially the centromedian and parafascicular nuclei). Although not portrayed in this figure, cortical inputs are topographically organized: association areas project mainly to the caudate nucleus, somatosensory and motor areas to the putamen, and limbic areas (including the hippocampus and amygdala) to the ventral striatum. The implication of these differing inputs, borne out by other aspects of basal ganglia connections and by behavioral studies, is that the different parts of the striatum have distinct functions.

Striatal efferents form the next stage in the path back to cerebral cortex by projecting to both segments of the globus pallidus and to the reticular part of the substantia nigra, which in most respects may be considered an extension of the globus pallidus.

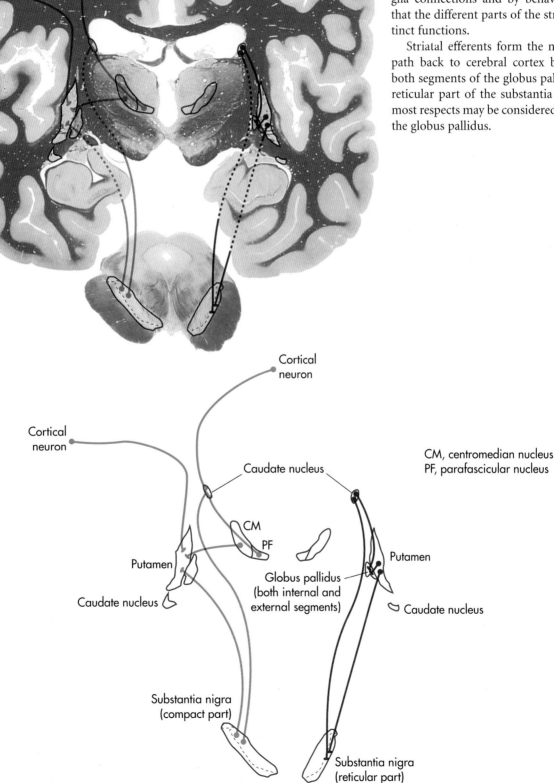

FIGURE 8-15
Connections of the globus pallidus; afferents on the left, efferents on the right. Excitatory connections are shown in green, inhibitory connections in red.

The globus pallidus is prominently subdivided over most of its extent into an external segment (adjacent to the putamen) and an internal segment. Both segments (as well as the reticular part of the substantia nigra, *SNr*) receive inputs from the striatum and the subthalamic nucleus. Afferents from the subthalamic nucleus penetrate the internal capsule as a series of small fiber bundles collectively called the subthalamic fasciculus.

The external *(GPe)* and internal *(GPi)* segments of the globus pallidus have distinct efferent projections. GPe projects to the subthalamic nucleus through the subthalamic fasciculus. GPi and SNr, in contrast, form the next stage in the path back to cerebral

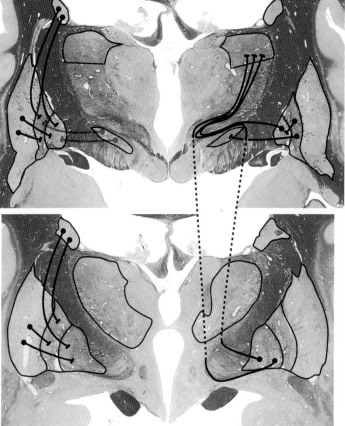

cortex, by projecting to the thalamus. Some efferents from GPi penetrate the internal capsule as a series of small fiber bundles collectively called the lenticular fasciculus; others emerge from the inferior surface of GPi and hook around the internal capsule in the ansa lenticularis. The ansa lenticularis and lenticular fasciculus join cerebellar efferents underneath the thalamus to form the thalamic fasciculus.

Although pallidal efferents in this figure are portrayed as ending in the ventral lateral nucleus, many actually end in the ventral anterior nucleus. Others reach more widespread thalamic sites (as might be expected in view of the striatal inputs from diverse cortical areas), such as the dorsomedial nucleus.

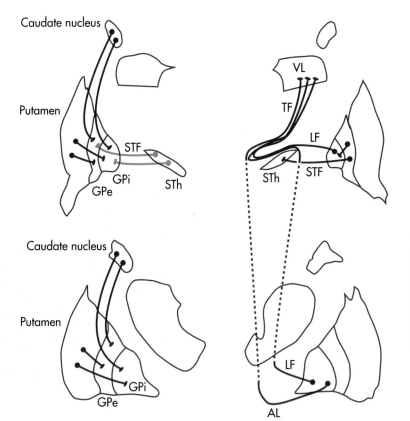

Abbreviations:
AL, ansa lenticularis
GPe, globus pallidus (external segment)
GPi, globus pallidus (internal segment)
LF, lenticular fasciculus
STF, subthalamic fasciculus
STh, subthalamic nucleus
TF, thalamic fasciculus
VL, ventral lateral nucleus of the thalamus

FIGURE 8-16
Connections of the substantia nigra. Excitatory connections are shown in green, inhibitory connections in red. (Projections from the compact part of the substantia nigra are shown in a third color because they excite some striatal neurons and inhibit others.) *(Histological section from Nolte J: The human brain, ed 4, St. Louis, 1999, Mosby.)*

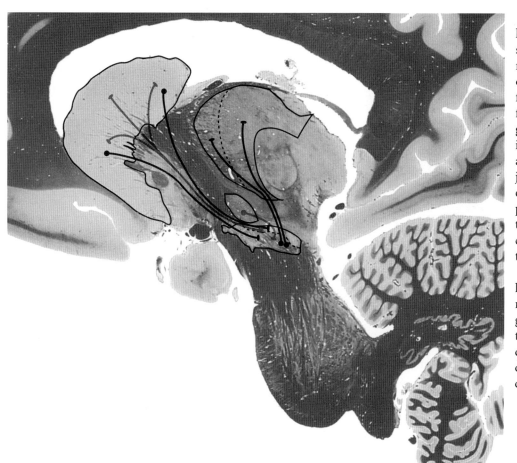

The substantia nigra is almost like two separate and distinct neural structures laminated together. The reticular part *(SNr)*, adjacent to the corticospinal and corticopontine fibers of the cerebral peduncle, is functionally a displaced part of the globus pallidus (internal segment): it receives inputs from the striatum and subthalamic nucleus and projects to the thalamus. (As in the case of the globus pallidus, its thalamic projections extend beyond the ventral anterior and ventral lateral nuclei, although this is not indicated in this figure.)

The compact part *(SNc)* is a collection of darkly pigmented neurons (from which the substantia nigra derives its name) that project to the striatum. These neurons release dopamine in the striatum, and their degeneration leads to Parkinson's disease.

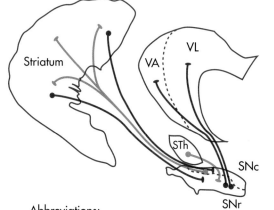

Abbreviations:
SNc, substantia nigra (compact part)
SNr, substantia nigra (reticular part)
STh, subthalamic nucleus
VA, ventral anterior nucleus of the thalamus
VL, ventral lateral nucleus of the thalamus

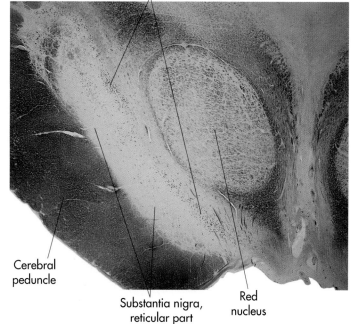

FIGURE 8-17
Connections of the subthalamic nucleus. Excitatory connections are
shown in green, inhibitory connections in red.

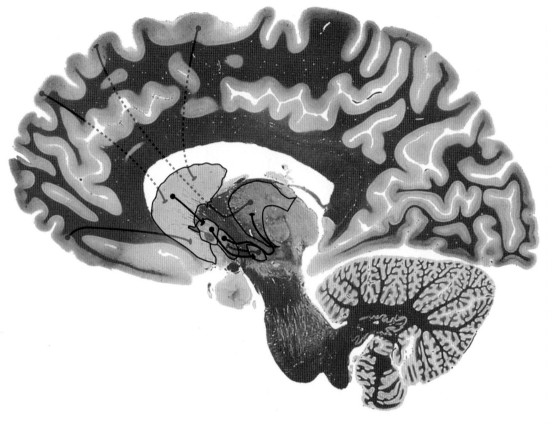

Despite its relatively small size, the subthalamic nucleus has surprisingly widespread connections, with inputs from the cerebral cortex (especially motor cortex) and interconnections with the thalamus, reticular formation, and several nuclei of the basal ganglia.

The most important of these connections from a functional standpoint may be inputs from the external segment of the globus pallidus and outputs to the internal segment of the globus pallidus (and to the reticular part of the substantia nigra). These form part of an indirect route through the basal ganglia (see inset below). One general strategy used by the basal ganglia may be to facilitate some cortical activities by signals conveyed in the direct route (described in Figure 8-13), while simultaneously suppressing competing cortical activities by means of signals in this indirect route.

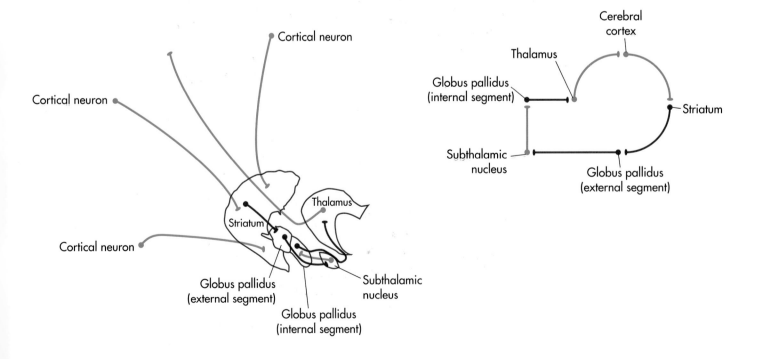

FIGURE 8-18
Gross anatomy of the cerebellum.

The cerebellum is even more highly convoluted than the cerebral hemispheres; this makes room for a large expanse of uniformly organized cerebellar cortex (see Figure 8-20). Its fissures are mostly oriented transversely, and prominent ones are used as landmarks to divide the cerebellum into lobes and lobules. Thus the very deep primary fissure separates the anterior and posterior lobes, and the posterolateral fissure separates the posterior and flocculonodular lobes.

Along lines roughly at right angles to the fissures, the entire cerebellum is divided into a narrow vermis that straddles the midline and a much larger hemisphere on each side.

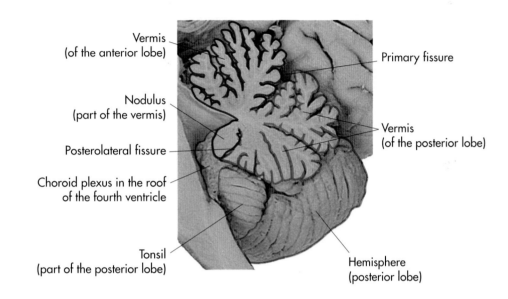

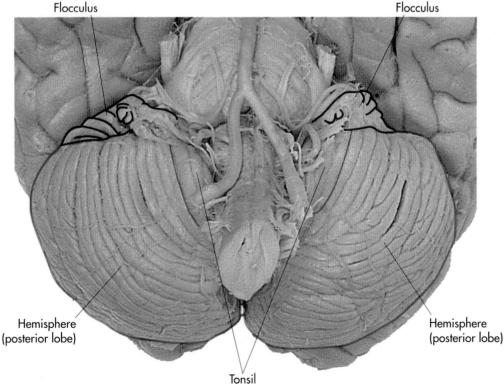

FIGURE 8-19
Routes into and out of the cerebellum: the cerebellar peduncles.

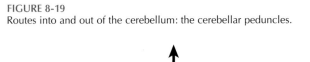

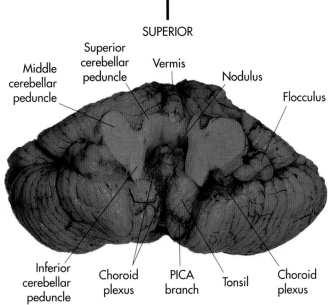

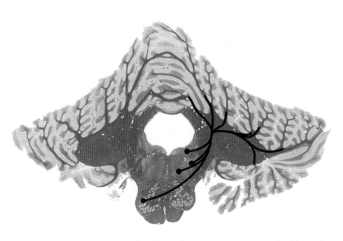

B, The inferior cerebellar peduncle is the major input route for fibers from the inferior olivary nucleus, vestibular nuclei, reticular formation, and spinal cord. (The inferior peduncle also contains some cerebellar efferents, particularly those bound for vestibular nuclei.)

A, Ventral surface of a cerebellum that had been removed from the brainstem by severing the cerebellar peduncles. The view is as if one were looking dorsally from the floor of the fourth ventricle toward its roof. *(From Nolte J:* The human brain, *ed 4, St. Louis, 1999, Mosby.)*

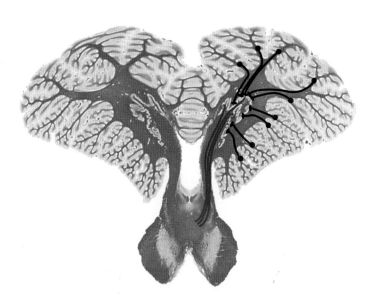

C, The middle cerebellar peduncle is the input route for information from cerebral cortex. Corticopontine fibers traverse the internal capsule and cerebral peduncle and terminate in pontine nuclei. Pontocerebellar fibers then project through the contralateral middle cerebellar peduncle to nearly all areas of the cerebellar cortex.

D, The superior cerebellar peduncle is the major output route from the cerebellum. Cerebellar cortex projects to a series of deep cerebellar nuclei, whose axons leave the cerebellum through this peduncle. (A few cerebellar afferents also travel through the superior peduncle.)

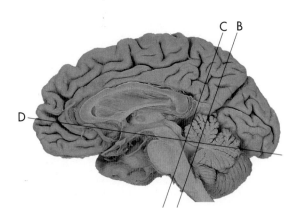

E, The planes of section shown in this figure. (The odd-looking section in *D* is part of Figure 6-5, *A* turned upside down so that its orientation more closely resembles that of *B* and *C*.)

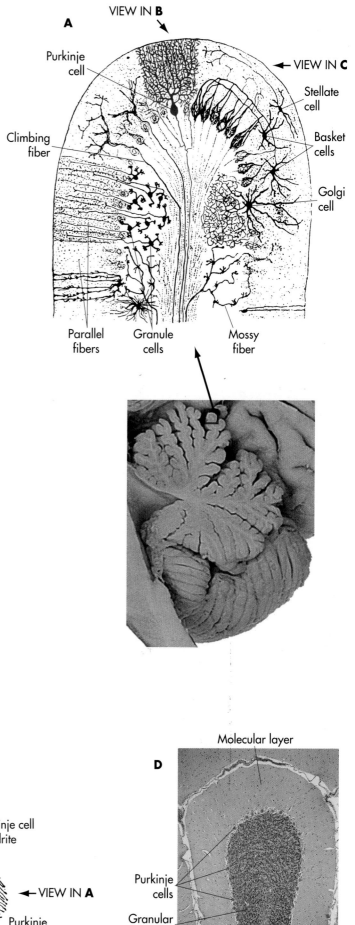

FIGURE 8-20

The structure of cerebellar cortex. **A,** Cross section of a single folium (as indicated in the inset). **B,** Oblique longitudinal section of a folium. **C,** Longitudinal section of a folium. **D,** Cross section of a single folium from a human cerebellum, stained with hematoxylin and eosin. *(A-C modified from Ramón y Cajal S: Histologie du système nerveux de l'homme et des vertébres, Paris, 1909–1911, Norbert Maloine. **D** courtesy of Dr. Nathaniel T. McMullen, Department of Cell Biology and Anatomy, The University of Arizona College of Medicine.)*

The lobes and lobules of the cerebellum are further subdivided by smaller sulci into a large number of folia. Each folium is covered by a remarkably uniform and precisely ordered cortex. Most of the various cell types contained in this cortex are indicated in *A*, but the basic organization is one in which two types of afferent fibers (mossy fibers and climbing fibers) enter the cortex and one type of axon (Purkinje cell axons) leaves to convey information to the deep cerebellar nuclei.

The climbing fibers all come from one place—the contralateral inferior olivary nucleus—and wrap around the proximal dendrites of Purkinje cells, forming powerful excitatory synapses.

All other cerebellar afferents enter the cerebellum as mossy fibers and terminate on the vast numbers of tiny granule cells in the granular layer. Granule cell axons ascend toward the cerebellar surface and bifurcate in the molecular layer to form parallel fibers, which run parallel to the long axis of a given folium. In so doing, the parallel fibers intersect the flattened, transversely oriented dendritic trees of Purkinje cells, where they make excitatory synapses.

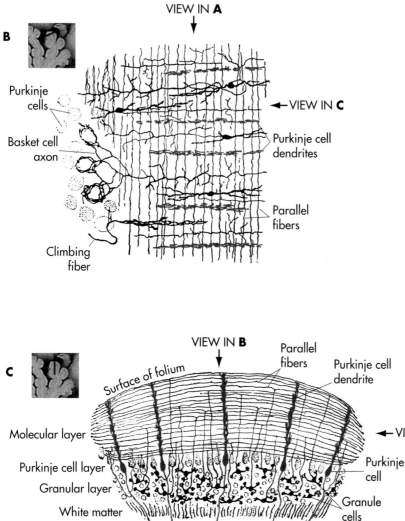

FIGURE 8-21
A, Afferents to the cerebellum.

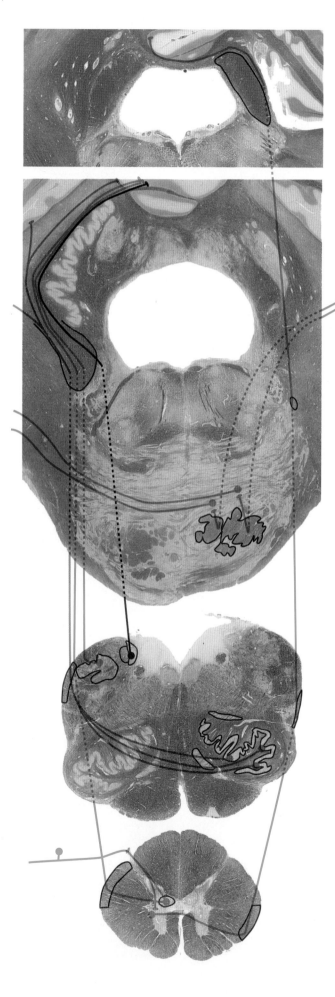

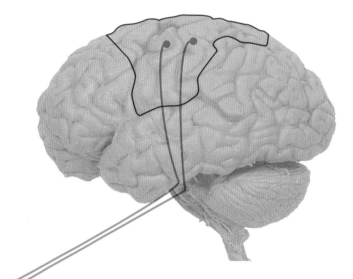

The cerebellum receives afferent inputs of three broad categories: afferents conveying information from the cerebral cortex, afferents conveying sensory information from a variety of subcortical sites, and climbing fibers from the contralateral inferior olivary nucleus.

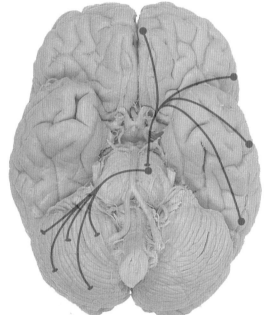

Cerebral cortical input (mostly, but not entirely, from motor and somatosensory areas) reaches the cerebellum through the middle cerebellar peduncle after a relay in the pontine nuclei. Most sensory information, arising most prominently in the spinal cord and vestibular nuclei, arrives via the inferior cerebellar peduncle (although a small amount traverses the superior peduncle). Axons leaving each inferior olivary nucleus travel through the contralateral inferior cerebellar peduncle before ending in the cerebellum as climbing fibers.

(The connections of the cerebellum are actually more widespread than this simple account would indicate, and it may have correspondingly broader functions. For example, interconnections between the cerebellum and the hypothalamus have been described, and the cerebellum may play a role in coordinating autonomic functions. Cortical inputs from association areas such as prefrontal cortex suggest that it may even be involved in higher cognitive functions.)

FIGURE 8-21, cont'd.
B, Afferents to the cerebellum, continued.

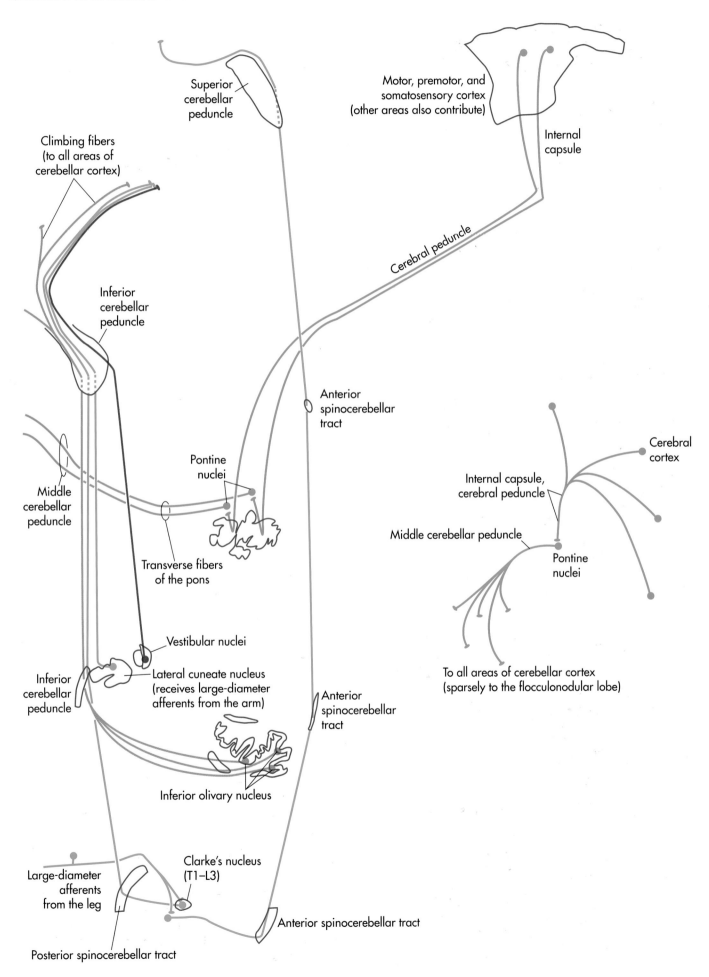

FIGURE 8-22
A, Efferents from the cerebellum to the cerebrum.

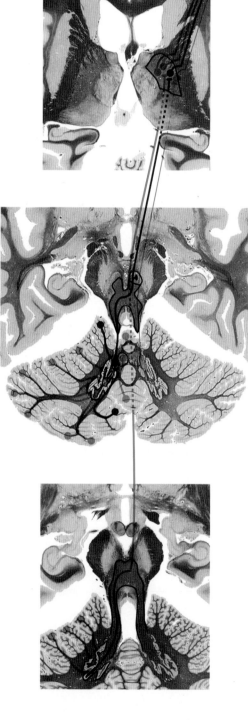

Purkinje cell axons are the sole output from cerebellar cortex. Some leave the cerebellum entirely, through the inferior cerebellar peduncle, to reach the vestibular nuclei. Most, however, project to a series of deep cerebellar nuclei in the roof of the fourth ventricle, which in turn provide most of the output from the cerebellum.

There are three deep cerebellar nuclei on each side, arranged in a lateral-to-medial sequence: the dentate, interposed,* and fastigial nuclei. This arrangement of the nuclei corresponds to three longitudinal zones of cerebellar cortex: the hemisphere most laterally, the vermis most medially, and an intermediate zone between the two. The pairing of deep nuclei and longitudinal zones of cortex is a reflection of functional subdivisions within the cerebellum that is also reflected in cerebellar outputs.

Each cerebellar hemisphere receives its major inputs from the cerebral cortex (motor, somatosensory, and other, more widespread areas) via pontine nuclei. Its outputs then influence the activity of motor and premotor cortex through a pathway involving the dentate nucleus and contralateral thalamus (primarily the ventral lateral nucleus). It is thought to play a role in planning skilled movements.

The intermediate zone receives information about the limbs from two major sources—motor cortex (via the pons) and the spinal cord (via spinocerebellar tracts). It is thus strategically positioned to compare intended and actual movements and to assist with moment-to-moment correction of movement, by way of connections with the interposed nucleus and motor cortex (via the thalamus).

The vermis receives information about axial muscles and body position from the vestibular nuclei and spinal cord and, through the fastigial nucleus, is involved in the maintenance and adjustment of posture. Most of this is accomplished at the level of the brainstem (see Figure 8-23), and the connections of the fastigial nucleus with the thalamus are relatively minor.

Finally, the flocculonodular lobe (which does not fit comfortably into this longitudinal zonation scheme) is critically involved in eye movements, by way of its connections with the vestibular nuclei.

---

*The interposed nucleus is itself a combination of the more lateral emboliform nucleus and more medial globose nucleus.

FIGURE 8-22, cont'd.
B, Efferents from the cerebellum to the cerebrum, continued. *(Histological section modified from Nolte J:* The human brain, *ed 4, St. Louis, 1999, Mosby.)*

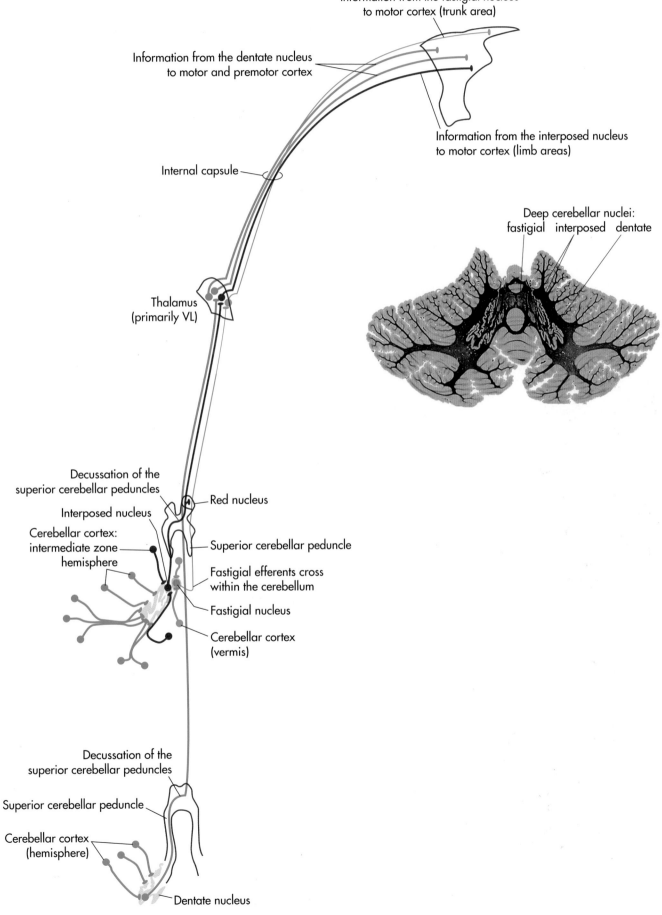

Information from the fastigial nucleus
to motor cortex (trunk area)

Information from the dentate nucleus
to motor and premotor cortex

Information from the interposed nucleus
to motor cortex (limb areas)

Internal capsule

Deep cerebellar nuclei:
fastigial   interposed   dentate

Thalamus
(primarily VL)

Decussation of the
superior cerebellar peduncles

Red nucleus

Interposed nucleus

Cerebellar cortex:
intermediate zone
hemisphere

Superior cerebellar peduncle

Fastigial efferents cross
within the cerebellum

Fastigial nucleus

Cerebellar cortex
(vermis)

Decussation of the
superior cerebellar peduncles

Superior cerebellar peduncle

Cerebellar cortex
(hemisphere)

Dentate nucleus

FIGURE 8-23
A, Efferents from the cerebellum to the brainstem.

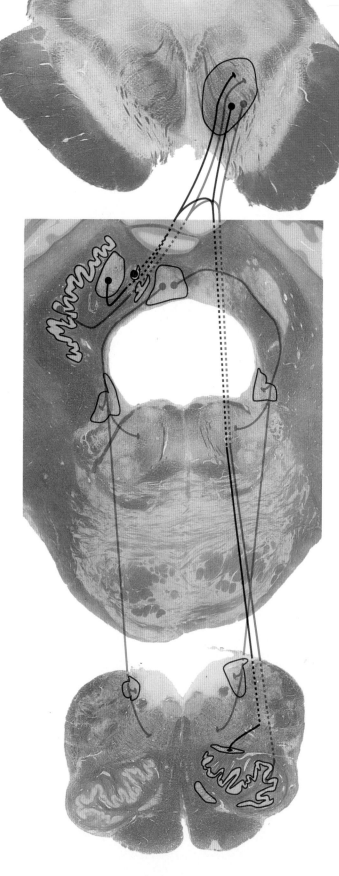

Each of the deep cerebellar nuclei also has outputs to sites in the brainstem; in the case of the fastigial nucleus these represent its major connections.

As the superior cerebellar peduncle passes through or around the red nucleus, some of its fibers (especially those from the interposed nucleus) synapse on rubral neurons. A relatively small part of the red nucleus gives rise to the rubrospinal tract, which decussates and proceeds to the spinal cord. This is one route through which the cerebellum helps make corrections to ongoing movements, but it is relatively unimportant in humans. Most neurons of the red nucleus project instead to the ipsilateral inferior olivary nucleus. In addition, some fibers leave the superior cerebellar peduncle as it traverses the brainstem, turn caudally, cross as the descending limb of the superior cerebellar peduncle, and reach the inferior olivary nucleus directly. The functional significance of these cerebellum–(red nucleus)–inferior olivary nucleus connections is not known with certainty, but they may play a role in motor learning.

The fastigial nucleus, consistent with its role in postural adjustments, projects bilaterally to the vestibular nuclei and reticular formation. Some of its efferents leave the cerebellum uncrossed through the inferior cerebellar peduncle. Others cross the midline within the cerebellum, hook over the top of the superior cerebellar peduncle (as the uncinate fasciculus), and join the contralateral inferior cerebellar peduncle.

FIGURE 8-23, cont'd.
B, Efferents from the cerebellum to the brainstem, continued.

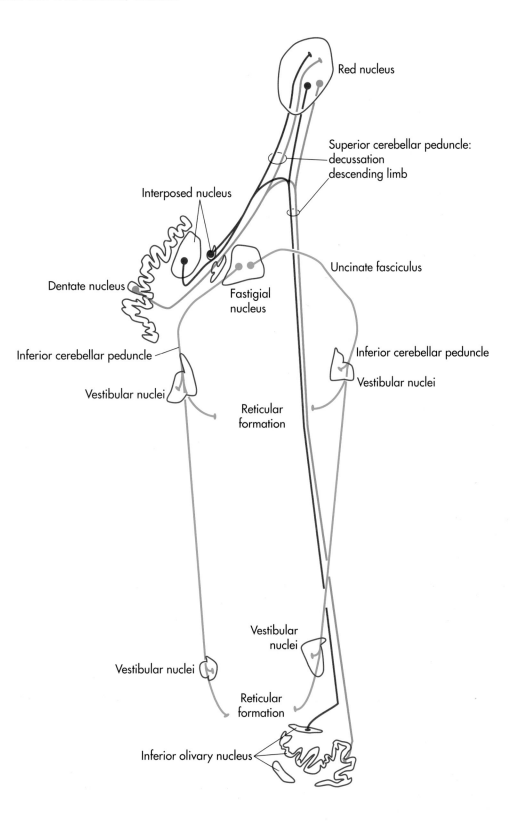

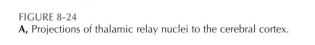

FIGURE 8-24

A, Projections of thalamic relay nuclei to the cerebral cortex.

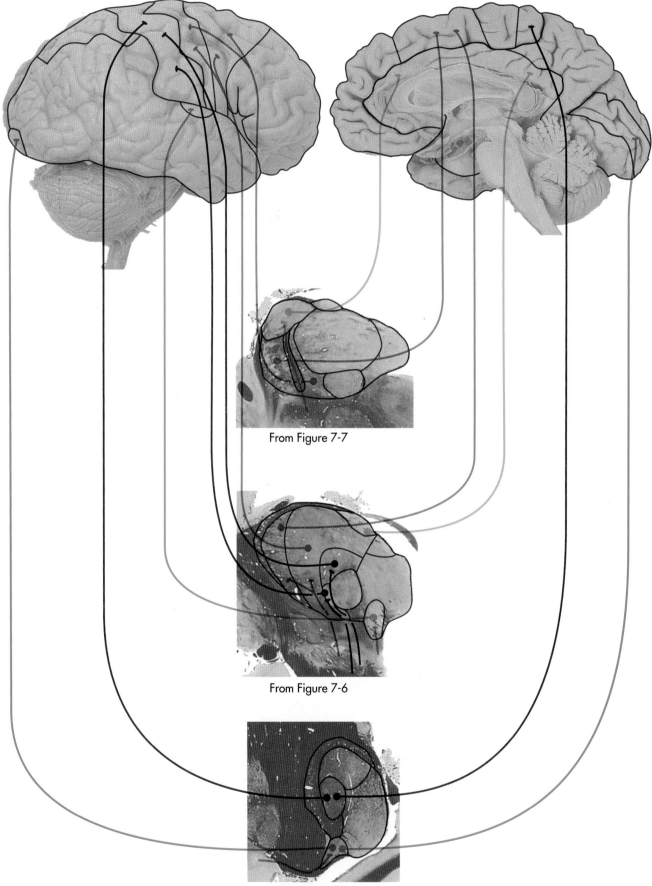

From Figure 7-7

From Figure 7-6

From Figure 7-5

FIGURE 8-24, cont'd.
B, Projections of thalamic relay nuclei to the cerebral cortex, continued (numbers = Brodmann's areas).

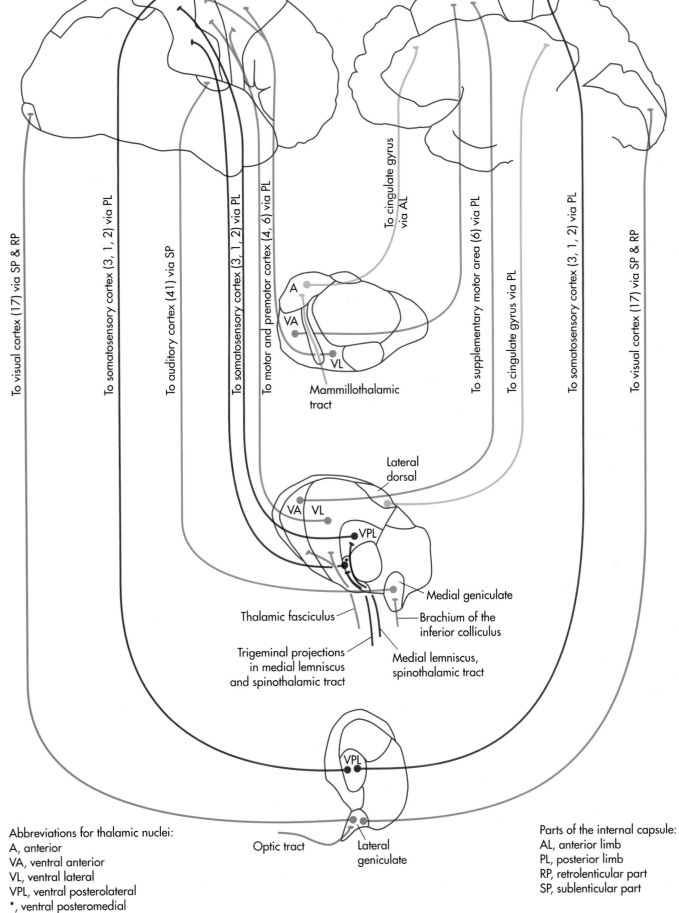

Abbreviations for thalamic nuclei:
A, anterior
VA, ventral anterior
VL, ventral lateral
VPL, ventral posterolateral
*, ventral posteromedial

Parts of the internal capsule:
AL, anterior limb
PL, posterior limb
RP, retrolenticular part
SP, sublenticular part

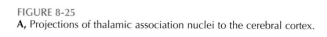

FIGURE 8-25

A, Projections of thalamic association nuclei to the cerebral cortex.

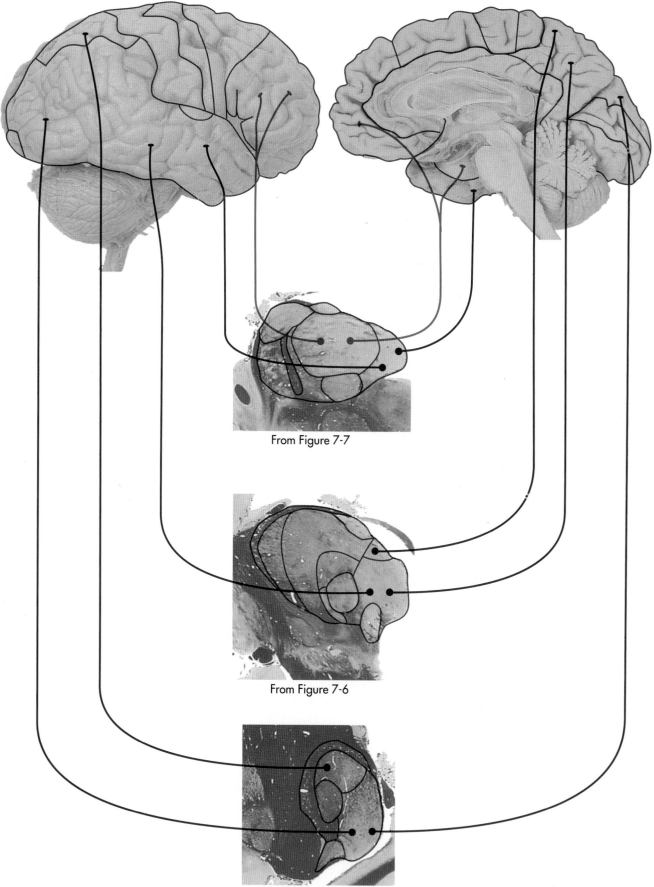

From Figure 7-7

From Figure 7-6

From Figure 7-5

FIGURE 8-25, cont'd.
B, Projections of thalamic association nuclei to the cerebral cortex, continued (numbers = Brodmann's areas).

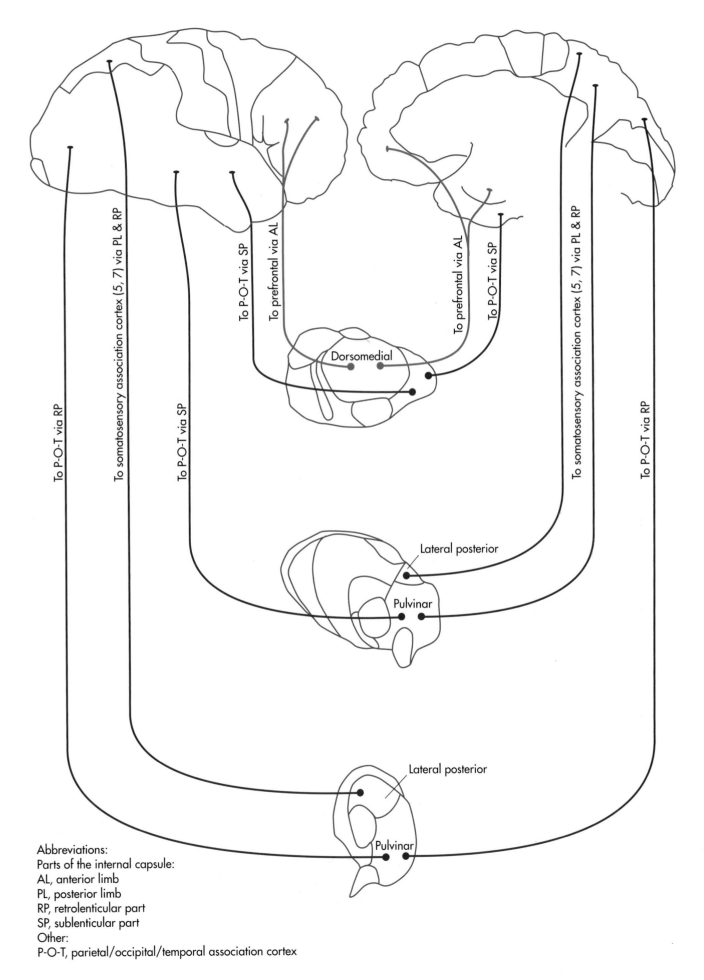

Abbreviations:
Parts of the internal capsule:
AL, anterior limb
PL, posterior limb
RP, retrolenticular part
SP, sublenticular part
Other:
P-O-T, parietal/occipital/temporal association cortex

FIGURE 8-26
A, The internal capsule.

2. The posterior limb and the retrolenticular and sublenticular parts of the internal capsule in coronal sections.

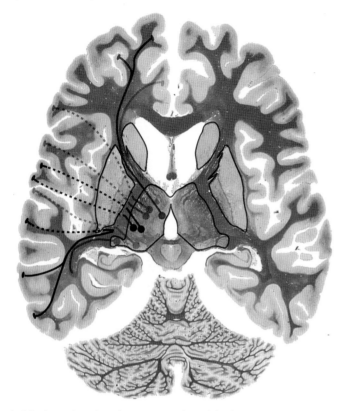

1. A horizontal section, demonstrating four of the five parts of the internal capsule.

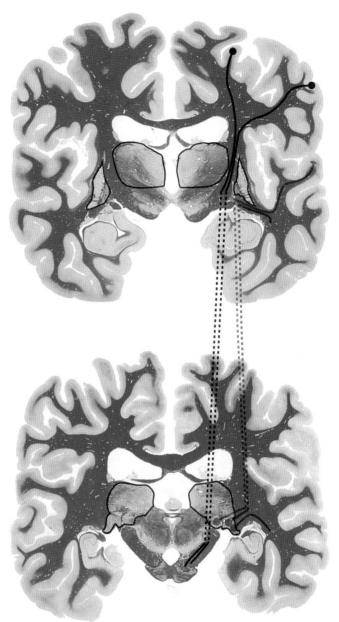

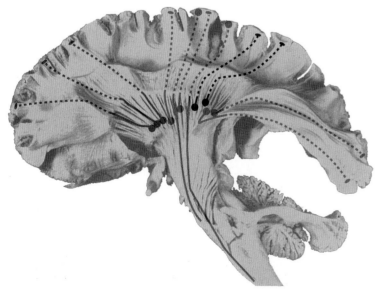

3. The entire internal capsule, shown in a dissection of the lateral surface of the brain. *(Modified from Ludwig E, Klingler J: Atlas cerebri humani, Boston, 1956, Little, Brown & Co.)*

The internal capsule is a compact bundle of fibers traveling to or from the cerebral cortex. Above the internal capsule the same fibers fan out within the hemisphere as the corona radiata; below it many of them continue on into the cerebral peduncle.

The internal capsule is shaped somewhat like an incomplete cone that partly surrounds the lenticular nucleus. Relationships between parts of the cone and the lenticular nucleus are used to define five regions: the anterior limb, between the lenticular nucleus and the head of the caudate nucleus; the posterior limb, between the lenticular nucleus and the thalamus; the genu, at the junction of the anterior and posterior limbs; the retrolenticular part, behind the lenticular nucleus; and the sublenticular part, dipping under the posterior end of the lenticular nucleus.

FIGURE 8-26, cont'd.
B, The internal capsule, continued.

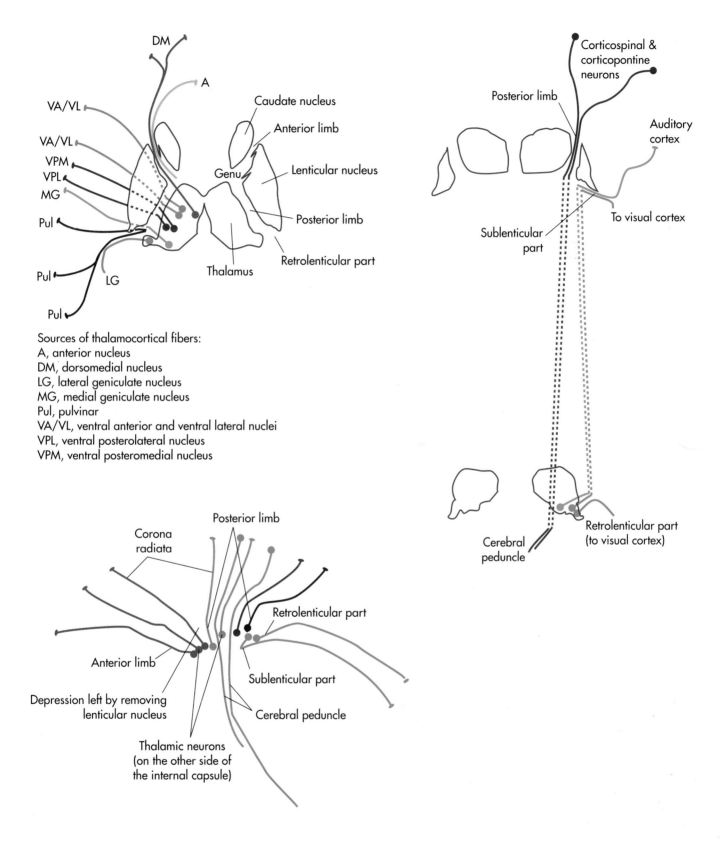

Sources of thalamocortical fibers:
A, anterior nucleus
DM, dorsomedial nucleus
LG, lateral geniculate nucleus
MG, medial geniculate nucleus
Pul, pulvinar
VA/VL, ventral anterior and ventral lateral nuclei
VPL, ventral posterolateral nucleus
VPM, ventral posteromedial nucleus

FIGURE 8-27
A, Afferents to the amygdala.

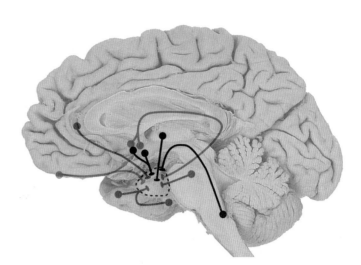

The amygdala, one of the major constituents of the limbic system, is a collection of nuclei underlying the uncus of the medial temporal lobe. It is centrally involved in assessing and remembering the emotional and drive-related significance of stimuli—deciding, for example, whether to flee from something or eat it. As such, it has widespread connections with the cerebral cortex, thalamus, hypothalamus, a variety of brainstem locations, and other sites. Inputs to the amygdala are summarized in the inset to the right, and indicated in more detail below.

Most amygdaloid afferents and efferents travel through two routes: (1) the stria terminalis, a long, curved bundle of fibers that travels in the wall of the lateral ventricle adjacent to the caudate nucleus, and (2) the ventral amygdalofugal pathway, a loosely organized group of fibers that pass underneath the lenticular nucleus on their way to and from the amygdala (a misleading name because this pathway contains both afferents and efferents). In addition, some afferents travel through the olfactory tract and others through the white matter of the temporal lobe.

FIGURE 8-27, cont'd.
B, Afferents to the amygdala, continued.

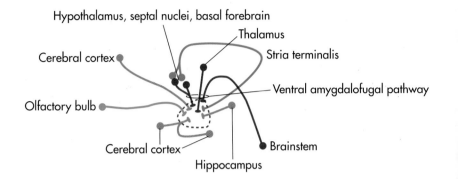

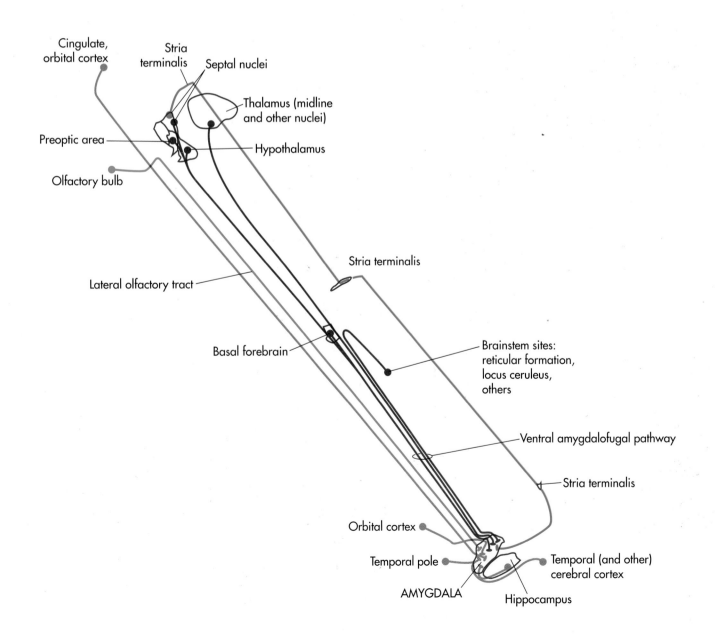

FIGURE 8-28
A, Efferents from the amygdala.

The efferents from the amygdala for the most part reciprocate its afferents, as indicated in the inset to the right and in more detail below. Efferents reach more widespread cortical areas than those in which afferents to the amygdala arise. In addition, efferents from the amygdala to the ventral striatum are presumed to play a role in initiating behavioral responses to emotionally significant stimuli.

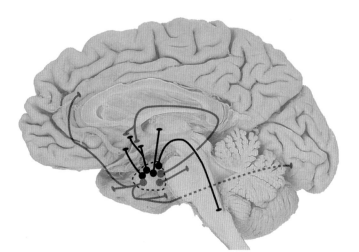

FIGURE 8-28, cont'd.
B, Efferents from the amygdala, continued.

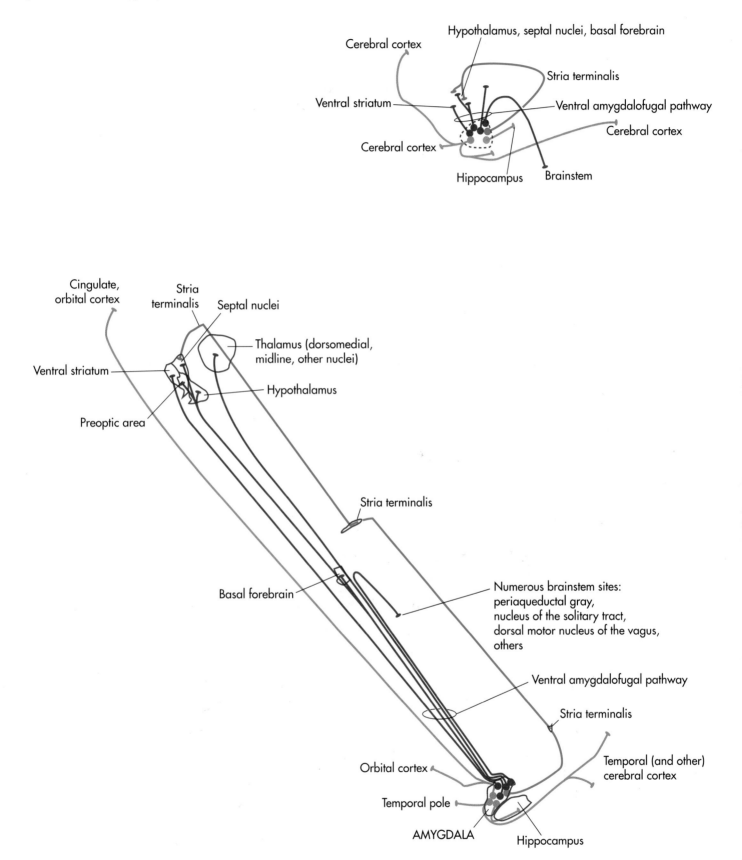

FIGURE 8-29
A, Afferents to the hippocampus.

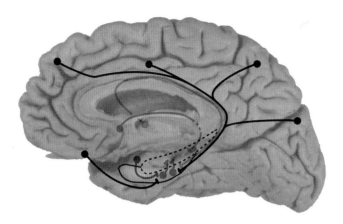

The hippocampus is a specialized area of cerebral cortex (see *C*)—conceptually, the edge of the cortical sheet—rolled into the medial temporal lobe. It extends in the wall of the lateral ventricle from an enlarged anterior end that overlaps the amygdala underneath the uncus to a tapering posterior end near the splenium of the corpus callosum.* Formally, it consists of the dentate gyrus, the hippocampus proper (also called *Ammon's horn* or *cornu ammonis*) and the subiculum, which merges with the cerebral cortex of the parahippocampal gyrus.

As in the case of the amygdala, the hippocampus is connected anatomically like a bridge between the diencephalon and widespread areas of cerebral cortex, in this case as the substrate for its critical role in consolidation of new cognitive memories.

Afferents from the hypothalamus and septal nuclei reach the hippocampus directly, but most others are relayed by adjacent parts of the parahippocampal gyrus (the entorhinal cortex). Many hippocampal afferents travel through either the cingulum, a curved fiber bundle underlying the cingulate gyrus, or the fornix, another curved fiber bundle that parallels the lateral ventricle. (The fornix is, however, primarily an efferent pathway.) To simplify this figure, various inputs are shown arriving at one specific part of the hippocampal complex, whereas in fact several project in parallel to multiple hippocampal elements (e.g., septal nuclei to dentate gyrus, hippocampus proper, and entorhinal cortex).

---

*The hippocampus actually continues over the top of the corpus callosum as a thin, apparently rudimentary, band of tissue—the indusium griseum, which is not indicated in this atlas. Hence the hippocampus, strictly defined, extends along the entire edge of the cortical mantle.

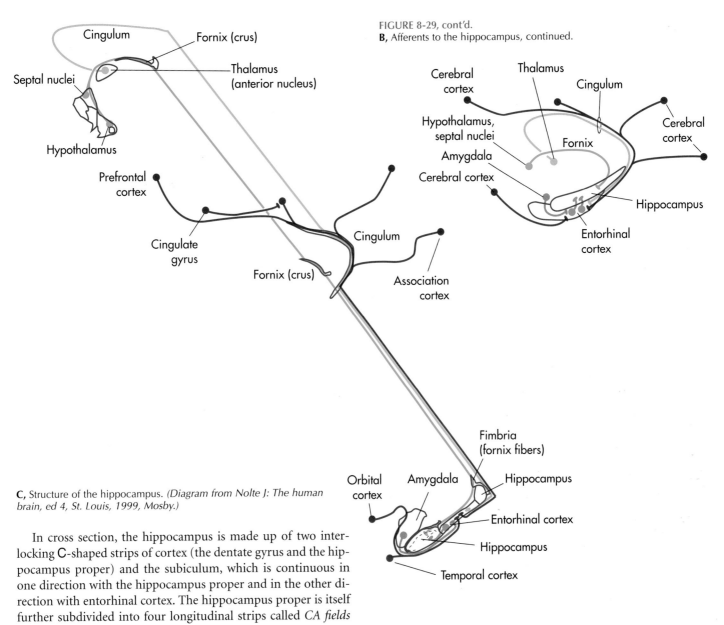

FIGURE 8-29, cont'd.
B, Afferents to the hippocampus, continued.

C, Structure of the hippocampus. *(Diagram from Nolte J: The human brain, ed 4, St. Louis, 1999, Mosby.)*

In cross section, the hippocampus is made up of two inter-locking C-shaped strips of cortex (the dentate gyrus and the hippocampus proper) and the subiculum, which is continuous in one direction with the hippocampus proper and in the other direction with entorhinal cortex. The hippocampus proper is itself further subdivided into four longitudinal strips called *CA fields* (*CA* for *cornu ammonis*).

The fundamental pattern of information flow in the hippocampus is unidirectional: afferents (mostly from entorhinal cortex) ➥ granule cells of the dentate gyrus ➥ CA3 pyramidal cells ➥ CA1 pyramidal cells ➥ pyramidal cells of the subiculum ➥ output targets. Thus most of the output of the hippocampus comes from the subiculum, although some comes from hippocampal pyramidal cells.

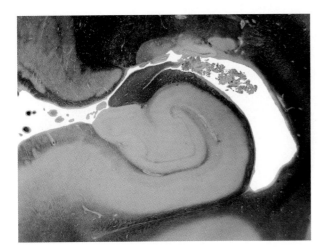

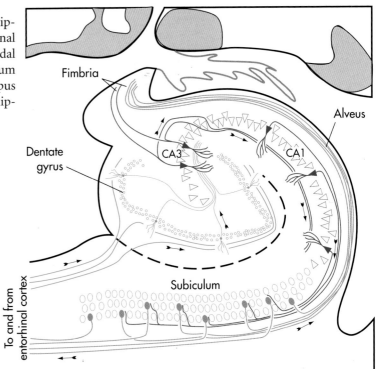

FIGURE 8-30
A, Efferents from the hippocampus.

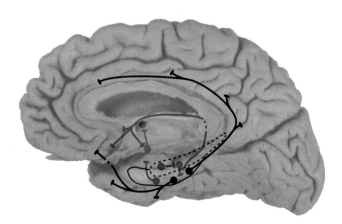

The anatomically most prominent efferent pathway from the hippocampus is the fornix, through which hippocampal pyramidal cells project to the septal nuclei and subicular neurons project to the septal nuclei, mammillary bodies, ventral striatum, and some cortical areas. The fornix is a long, curved tract that starts out as fibers (the alveus) on the ventricular surface of the hippocampus proper. These fibers merge into the fimbria (literally "the fringe" of the hippocampus), which parts company with the dwindling hippocampus near the splenium of the corpus callosum and emerges from the temporal lobe as the crus of the fornix. The crus then approaches its counterpart from the other hemisphere and continues traveling anteriorly, adjacent to the midline and at the inferior edge of the septum pellucidum, as the

body of the fornix. At the level of the interventricular foramen, fornix fibers begin to splay out as they move toward their final destinations. Some pass in front of the anterior commissure (the precommissural fornix) to reach the septal nuclei and parts of the frontal lobe. Others turn posteriorly and end directly in the anterior nucleus of the thalamus. A large number descend through the hypothalamus in the column of the fornix, mostly directed toward the mammillary body.

Large numbers of subicular efferents, however, bypass the fornix and project directly to the amygdala, entorhinal cortex, and other cortical areas. (This is presumably part of the reason why bilateral damage to the hippocampus causes a much more severe memory deficit than does bilateral damage to the fornix.) As in the case of afferents to the hippocampus, more than one hippocampal component may project in parallel to the same structure (e.g., both subiculum and entorhinal cortex to the amygdala).

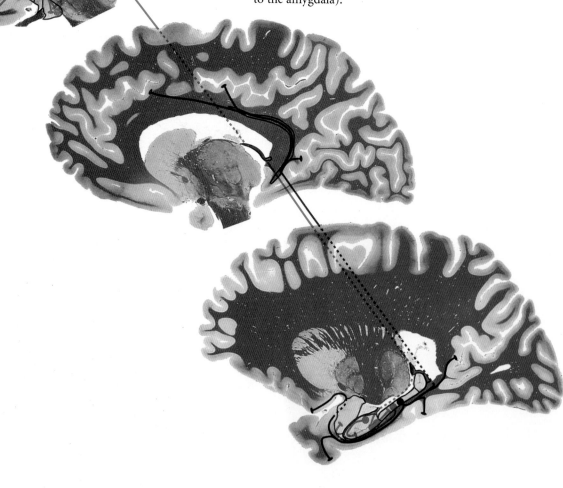

FIGURE 8-30, cont'd.
B, Efferents from the hippocampus, continued.

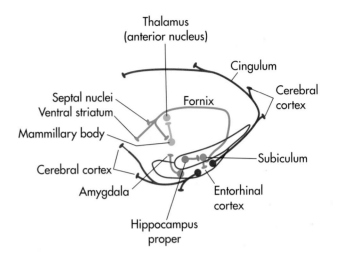

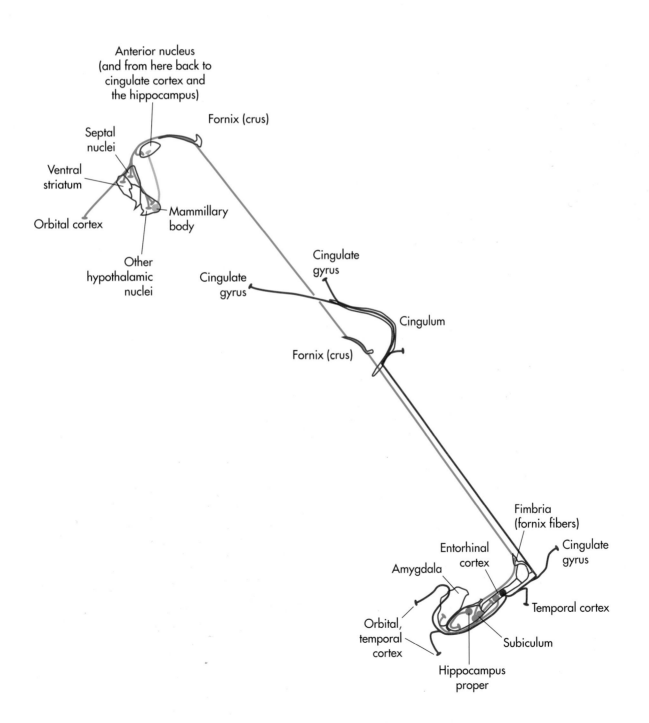

FIGURE 8-31
Neurons and pathways that use acetylcholine as a neurotransmitter.

Some neurotransmitters are found in neurons widely distributed in the nervous system. Glutamate, for example, is a common transmitter used by neurons throughout the brain at excitatory synapses. Similarly, gamma-aminobutyric acid (GABA) is a nearly ubiquitous transmitter used at inhibitory synapses. In contrast, some transmitters are found only in neurons in restricted locations (although the axons of these neurons may be distributed widely). Acetylcholine, the first neurotransmitter to be discovered, is a case in point.

Acetylcholine is of major importance in the peripheral nervous system, where it is the principal transmitter released by motor neurons, preganglionic autonomic neurons, postganglionic parasympathetic neurons, and some postganglionic sympathetic neurons. Within the brain, its distribution is more restricted. Acetylcholine is used as a neurotransmitter by some interneurons of the striatum and by some parts of the reticular formation. However, the most prominent collection of cholinergic neurons in the brain is found in the basal nucleus (of Meynert), the septal nuclei, and nearby parts of the basal forebrain. Collectively, these neurons project through the cingulum and the external capsule (the white matter between the claustrum and the lenticular nucleus) and blanket the cerebral cortex and amygdala with cholinergic endings. In addition, some of the septal neurons send cholinergic axons through the fornix to the hippocampus.

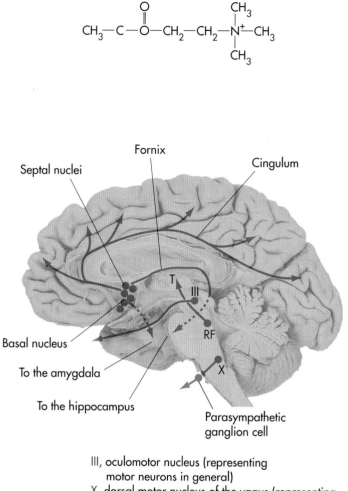

III, oculomotor nucleus (representing motor neurons in general)
X, dorsal motor nucleus of the vagus (representing preganglionic autonomic neurons in general)
RF, reticular formation
T, thalamus

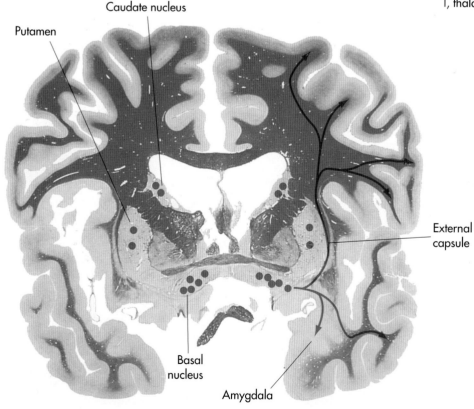

FIGURE 8-32
Neurons and pathways that use norepinephrine as a neurotransmitter.

Norepinephrine, one of the catecholamine neurotransmitters (so called because of the catechol group, shown in red, that forms part of the molecule), is the transmitter used by most postganglionic sympathetic neurons. Within the CNS it is found in a series of pontine and medullary neurons with long, branching axons that collectively innervate most areas of the brain and spinal cord.

The majority of these noradrenergic neurons (noradrenaline is a synonym for norepinephrine) are located in the locus ceruleus, a column of pigmented cells in the rostral pons (see Figure 3-11). Others are located in the dorsal motor nucleus of the vagus, the nucleus of the solitary tract, the medullary reticular formation, and a few other sites.

Ascending noradrenergic fibers (mostly from the locus ceruleus) travel through the brainstem in the dorsal longitudinal fasciculus and central tegmental tract. When they reach the cerebrum, many of them join the medial forebrain bundle, which travels longitudinally through the lateral hypothalamus. They then diverge to innervate practically all cerebral areas. Descending noradrenergic fibers (many from more caudally located neurons) similarly diverge to innervate the cerebellum, brainstem, and spinal cord.

These diffuse, nearly global projections are clearly unsuitable for mediating functions that depend on precise, point-to-point communication, and it is thought that instead they are involved in regulating the overall level of activity in the brain (e.g., as levels of attention and vigilance vary).

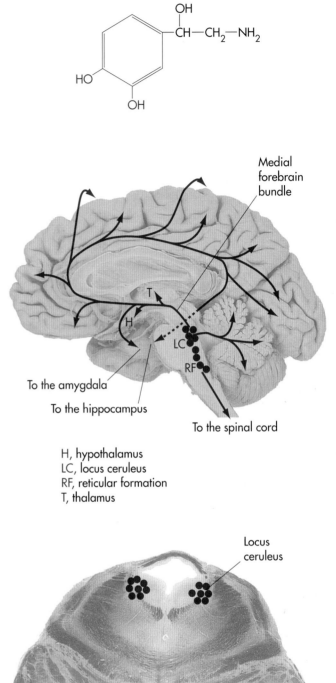

Medial forebrain bundle

To the amygdala

To the hippocampus

To the spinal cord

H, hypothalamus
LC, locus ceruleus
RF, reticular formation
T, thalamus

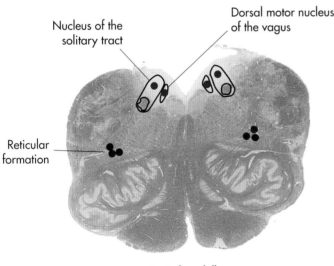

Nucleus of the solitary tract

Dorsal motor nucleus of the vagus

Reticular formation

Rostral medulla

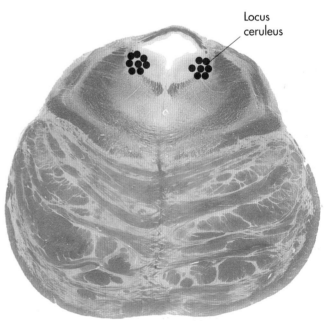

Locus ceruleus

Rostral pons

FIGURE 8-33
Neurons and pathways that use dopamine as a neurotransmitter.

Dopamine is a second major catecholamine neurotransmitter (so called because of the catechol group, shown in red, that forms part of the molecule). Most dopaminergic neurons are located in the midbrain, either in the substantia nigra (compact part) or in the medially adjacent ventral tegmental area. They project rostrally to most parts of the cerebrum, in three partially overlapping streams of fibers.

The first of these streams is the projection from the substantia nigra (compact part) to the caudate nucleus and putamen (see Figure 8-14). Because of its origin in the midbrain, this nigrostriatal pathway is also referred to as the mesostriatal dopaminergic pathway (midbrain = mesencephalon).

Mesolimbic and mesocortical fibers originate mainly in the ventral tegmental area and project through the medial forebrain bundle to limbic-related subcortical structures (such as the amygdala, septal nuclei, and ventral striatum) and to cerebral cortex (especially motor and limbic areas).

Additional dopaminergic neurons are found in the retina and in the hypothalamus. The latter project to the infundibular stalk, where dopamine released into capillaries of the pituitary portal system regulates the secretion of prolactin by the anterior pituitary.

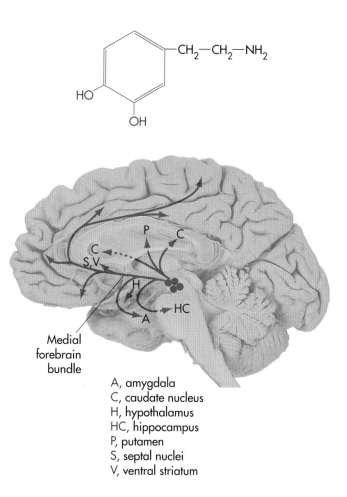

Medial
forebrain
bundle

A, amygdala
C, caudate nucleus
H, hypothalamus
HC, hippocampus
P, putamen
S, septal nuclei
V, ventral striatum

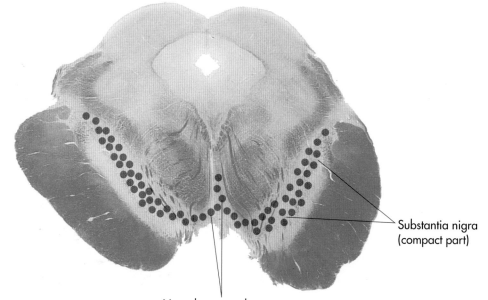

Substantia nigra
(compact part)

Ventral tegmental area

FIGURE 8-34
Neurons and pathways that use serotonin as a neurotransmitter.

Serotonin (shown below), a derivative of tryptophan, is used as a neurotransmitter by a collection of neurons located at most brainstem levels in a series of raphe* nuclei. Serotoninergic neurons, like noradrenergic neurons, give rise to widely branched axons that innervate most parts of the CNS, including the hypothalamus *(H)*, striatum *(S)*, and thalamus *(T)*. Serotonin, like norepinephrine, is thought to be involved in regulating the overall level of activity in the brain.

*The Greek word *rhaphe* means "seam" and is used in this case to refer to the midline seam between the two halves of the brainstem.

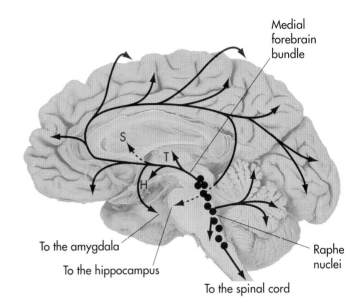

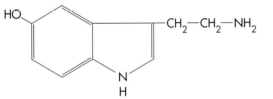

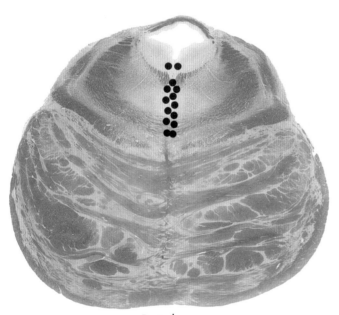

Rostral pons

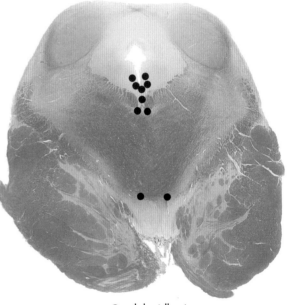

Caudal midbrain

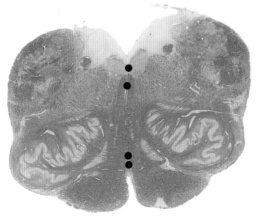

Rostral medulla

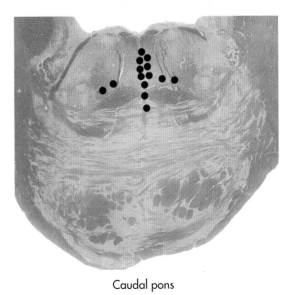

Caudal pons

CLINICAL IMAGING*

For many decades, the central nervous systems of living individuals could be examined only indirectly, for example by using x-rays to study changes in the bones surrounding the CNS or the blood vessels around or within it. In addition, these imaging studies involved projecting all the x-ray density under investigation in the head (a three-dimensional structure) onto a two-dimensional sheet of film. As a result, the images of structures actually separated in space (e.g., the middle cerebral and anterior cerebral branches in Figure 9-17) are superimposed on each other in these studies.

Recent years have seen revolutionary changes in clinical imaging, partly a result of the use of computers to reconstruct two-dimensional "slices" at various levels of a patient's head (i.e., tomography) and partly a result of the ability to construct images based on parameters other than x-ray density.

The most commonly used clinical imaging techniques at present are x-ray computed tomography (CT) and magnetic resonance (MR). CT provides images based on x-ray density, so structures that attenuate x-rays, such as bone, appear light; areas filled with air or cerebrospinal fluid, which do not attenuate x-rays as much, appear much darker. Appropriate techniques can accentuate brain, bone, or blood (Figures 9-1 to 9-3). MR (Figure 9-4), in contrast, provides images based on chemical concentrations (most commonly emphasizing the concentration of free water). This chapter provides a series of examples of the use of CT and MR in clinical imaging. In addition, because traditional angiographic techniques still yield the most highly detailed images of the cerebral vasculature, examples of angiograms are provided as well.

---

*With the assistance of Robert B. Handy, MD and images provided by Raymond Carmody, MD and Joachim F. Seeger, MD.

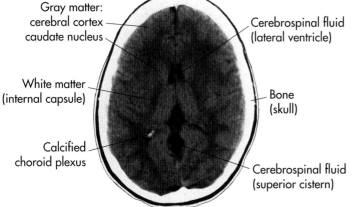

FIGURE 9-1
A horizontal (axial) CT scan, demonstrating the relative x-ray densities of cranial structures. The computer was adjusted so that the middle of the gray scale corresponds to the x-ray density of brain. Hence bone is white, fluid is black, and gray and white matter can be differentiated.

FIGURE 9-2
A horizontal (axial) CT scan, adjusted so that the gray scale corresponds to the x-ray density of bone. Air (and fluid) are black. Little soft-tissue detail can be seen, but the details and relative densities of different bones (e.g., sphenoid versus temporal) are apparent.

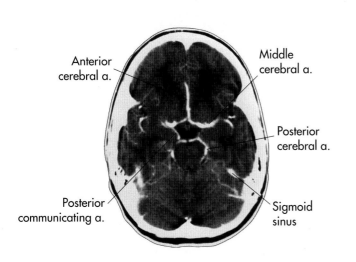

FIGURE 9-3
Blood (typically in blood vessels) can be seen more easily if an iodinated, x-ray dense contrast agent is injected intravenously before to the CT scan.

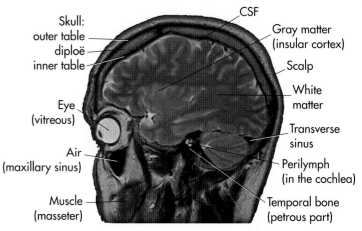

FIGURE 9-4
A parasagittal MR image. The concentration of water ranges from very low (air, bone) to intermediate levels (brain, muscle) to very high (cerebrospinal fluid, perilymph), allowing all of these to be differentiated. (The appearance of blood vessels is explained later.)

FIGURE 9-5
A series of seven CT images at different levels of a normal brain.

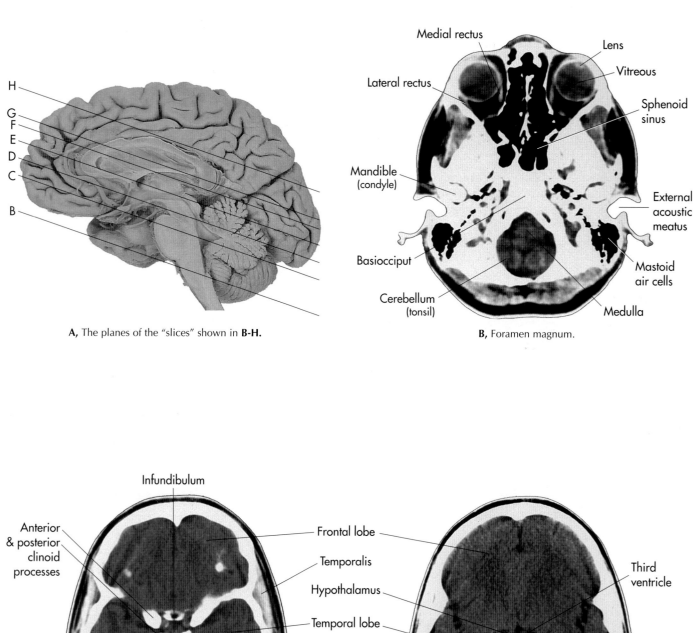

H
G
F
E
D
C
B

A, The planes of the "slices" shown in **B-H.**

Medial rectus
Lens
Vitreous
Lateral rectus
Sphenoid sinus
Mandible (condyle)
External acoustic meatus
Basiocciput
Mastoid air cells
Cerebellum (tonsil)
Medulla

B, Foramen magnum.

Infundibulum

Anterior & posterior clinoid processes
Frontal lobe
Temporalis
Hypothalamus
Temporal lobe
Lateral ventricle (inferior horn)
Cerebral peduncle
Fourth ventricle
Mastoid air cells
Basal pons
Cerebellum: hemisphere vermis

Third ventricle
Uncus
Ambient cistern

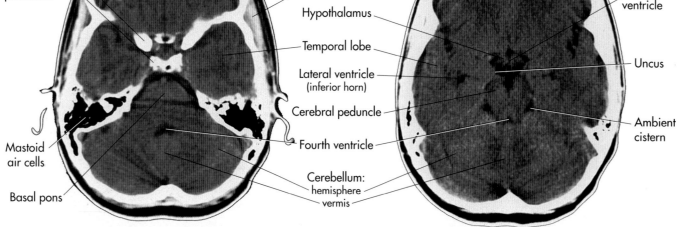

C, Pituitary gland and fourth ventricle. (The streaks cutting across the cerebellum and pons are artifacts resulting from the presence of dense bone nearby. The density in each frontal lobe results from nearby bone in the orbital roofs.)

D, Base of the diencephalon.

FIGURE 9-5, cont'd.
Normal CT images.

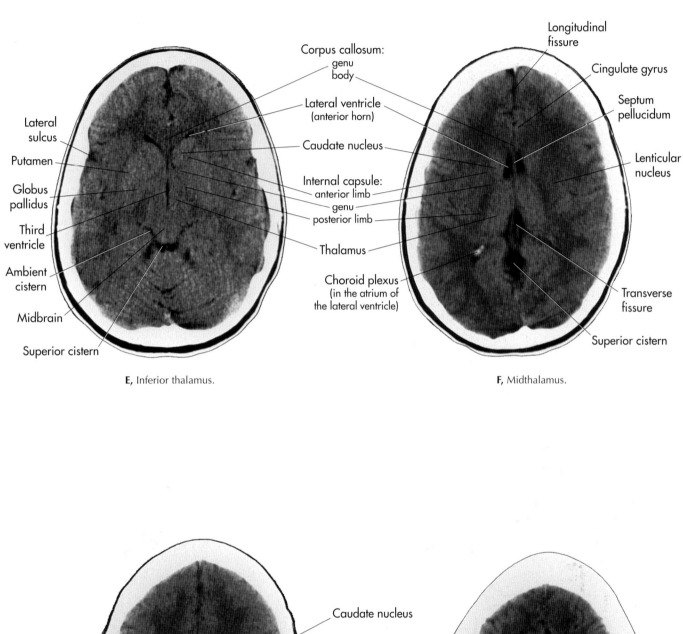

Corpus callosum:
  genu
  body

Lateral ventricle
(anterior horn)

Caudate nucleus

Internal capsule:
  anterior limb
  genu
  posterior limb

Thalamus

Choroid plexus
(in the atrium of
the lateral ventricle)

Lateral
sulcus

Putamen

Globus
pallidus

Third
ventricle

Ambient
cistern

Midbrain

Superior cistern

Longitudinal
fissure

Cingulate gyrus

Septum
pellucidum

Lenticular
nucleus

Transverse
fissure

Superior cistern

E, Inferior thalamus.

F, Midthalamus.

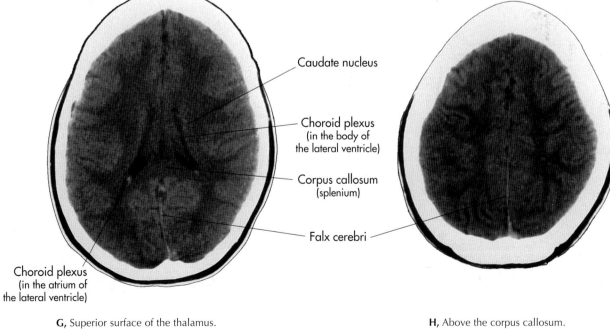

Caudate nucleus

Choroid plexus
(in the body of
the lateral ventricle)

Corpus callosum
(splenium)

Falx cerebri

Choroid plexus
(in the atrium of
the lateral ventricle)

G, Superior surface of the thalamus.

H, Above the corpus callosum.

FIGURE 9-6
A series of seven CT images from the same patient shown in Figure 9-5. In this case an iodinated intravenous contrast agent was administered before the CT study, making blood vessels visible.

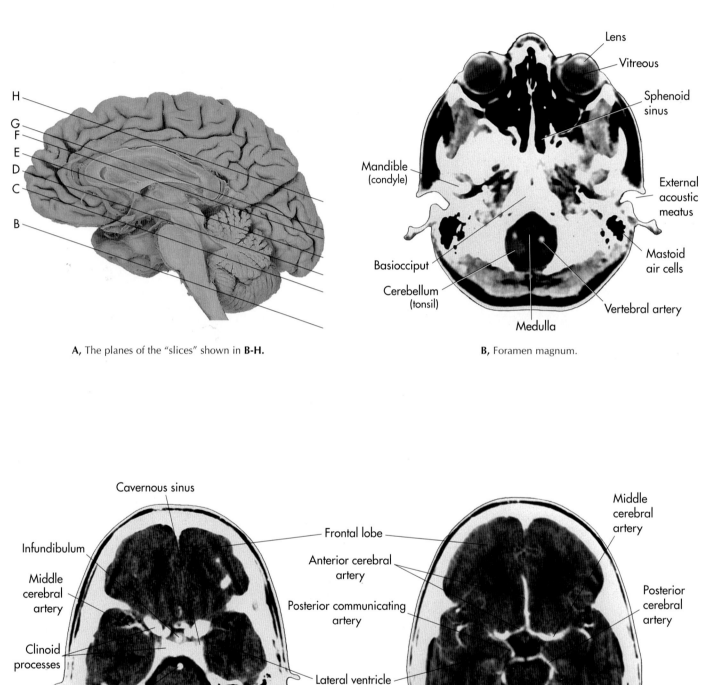

A, The planes of the "slices" shown in B-H.

B, Foramen magnum.

C, Cavernous sinus.

D, Circle of Willis.

FIGURE 9-6, cont'd.
Contrasted CT images.

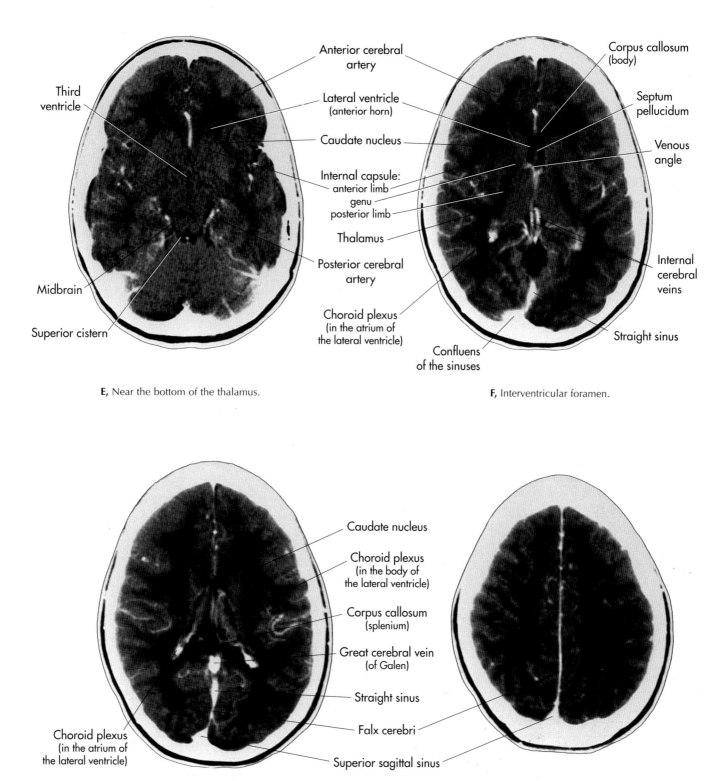

E, Near the bottom of the thalamus.

F, Interventricular foramen.

G, Superior surface of the thalamus.

H, Above the corpus callosum.

FIGURE 9-7
The use of CT to demonstrate intracranial pathology.

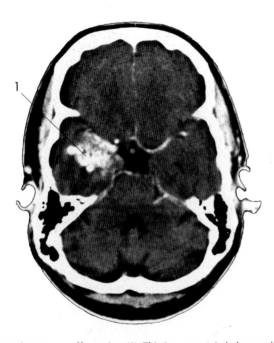

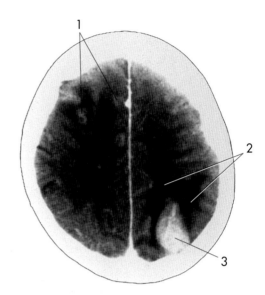

A, An arteriovenous malformation *(1)*. This is a congenital abnormality consisting of a tangle of enlarged vessels connecting the arterial and venous systems, here made visible by an intravenous iodinated contrast agent.

B, Several metastatic tumors near junctions between gray and white matter *(1, 3)*. The blood-brain barrier breaks down in such tumors, allowing iodinated contrast agent to leak out. The dark area *(2)* is edema surrounding the largest tumor.

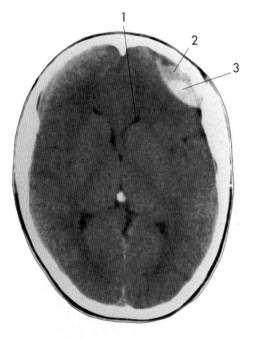

C, An epidural hematoma resulting from a skull fracture and torn meningeal artery. As the patient remained supine, red blood cells settled to the bottom of the hematoma, giving it a divided appearance *(2, 3)*. The expanding pool of blood compressed the anterior horn of the left lateral ventricle *(1)* and shifted the left half of the brain toward the right.

D, The same patient shown in *C,* but with CT parameters set to show bone detail. Now the skull fracture *(1)* is visible, as well as contused and swollen tissue *(2)* at the site of injury.

CT reconstructs images based on spatial variations in x-ray density, so the relatively small density differences between gray and white matter limit its ability to differentiate between different areas of the brain. In addition, the much greater x-ray density of bone can overwhelm these small gray-white differences and cause artifacts in bony areas such as the posterior fossa (see Figure 9-5, C).

MR imaging overcomes these problems by being exquisitely sensitive to spatial variations in the concentration and physicochemical situation of particular atomic nuclei (almost always hydrogen nuclei). Nuclei with an odd number of protons or neutrons, such as hydrogen nuclei, behave like tiny magnets. Imposing a powerful magnetic field on something containing these nuclei (e.g., someone's head) causes a net tendency for the nuclei to align themselves with the external field. Once so aligned, the nuclei preferentially absorb and then emit electromagnetic energy at a particular frequency (the resonant frequency for that nucleus in that situation). Hence applying radio-frequency pulses to a subject in a strong, static magnetic field and then measuring the spatial distributions of various time constants with which the absorbed energy is re-emitted can provide the data for construction of images based on different tissue properties.

Two time constants—T1 and T2—are important in clinical imaging. T1 is the time constant with which nuclei return to alignment with the static field. T2 is the time constant with which nuclei, all perturbed at the same time by radiofrequency pulses, lose alignment with each other. T1- and T2-weighted images emphasize different tissue parameters in different ways (Figure 9-8); T2-weighted images, for example, are highly sensitive to small changes in water concentration and so are very useful for demonstrating pathology within the brain. A series of reverse-contrast T2-weighted images (Figures 9-9 and 9-10) is used in Figures 9-11 through 9-13 to show the extraordinary anatomical detail that can be demonstrated by MR imaging.

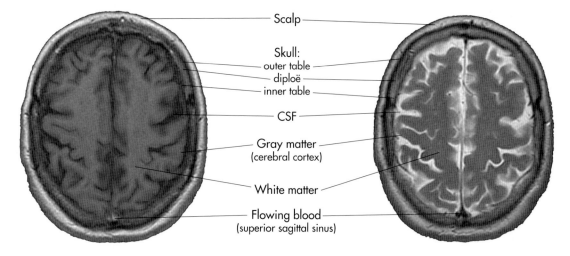

Scalp

Skull:
outer table
diploë
inner table

CSF

Gray matter
(cerebral cortex)

White matter

Flowing blood
(superior sagittal sinus)

FIGURE 9-8
In T1-weighted images *(left),* white matter is lighter than gray matter and CSF is dark. Conversely, in T2-weighted images *(right),* white matter is darker than gray matter and CSF is bright and prominent. In both, air and dense bone, which contain relatively few hydrogen nuclei, are dark. The appearance of flowing blood depends on a number of technical parameters, but in many instances (such as the T2 image on the right) perturbed nuclei have left the area before the imaging measurement is made, so the blood vessel appears dark, as though no hydrogen nuclei were present.

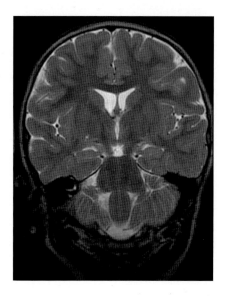

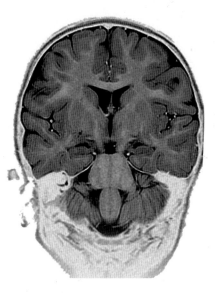

FIGURE 9-9
The T2-weighted coronal slice that forms the basis for Figure 9-11, *E.*

FIGURE 9-10
After reversing the contrast in Figure 9-9, gray matter looks gray, white matter looks white, and cerebrospinal fluid (in ventricles and subarachnoid space) looks black. Bone, air, and flowing blood look white. This contrast reversal of T2-weighted images was used in Figures 9-11 to 9-13.

FIGURE 9-11
Coronal MR images, T2 weighted, contrast reversed.

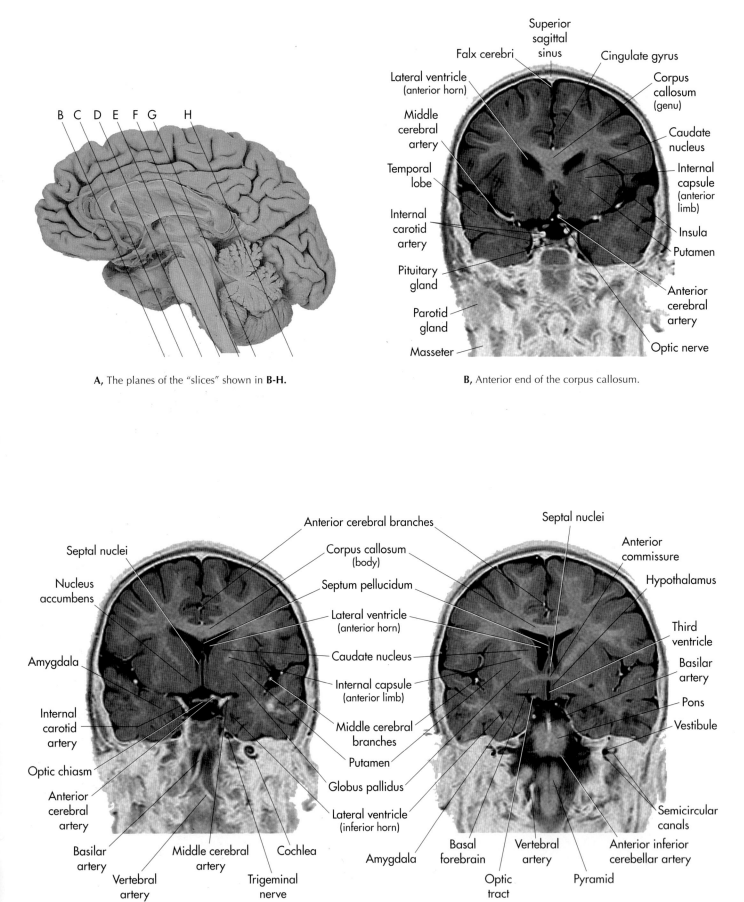

A, The planes of the "slices" shown in **B-H.**

B, Anterior end of the corpus callosum.

C, Optic chiasm.

D, Anterior commissure.

FIGURE 9-11, cont'd.
Coronal MR images, T2 weighted, contrast reversed.

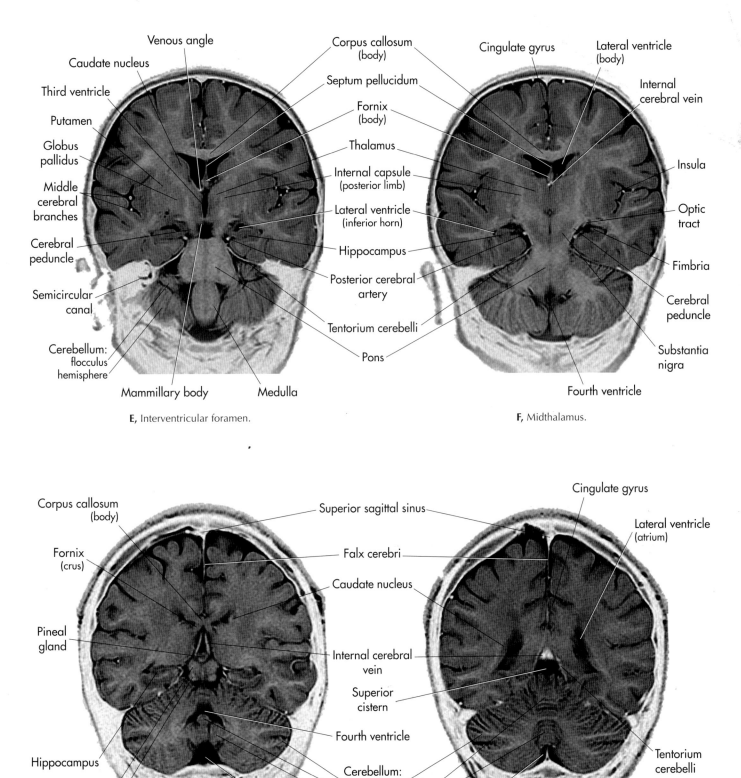

E, Interventricular foramen.

F, Midthalamus.

G, Posterior thalamus.

H, Splenium of the corpus callosum.

FIGURE 9-12
Axial (horizontal) MR images, T2 weighted, contrast reversed. This patient had an unusually (but not abnormally) large cisterna magna.

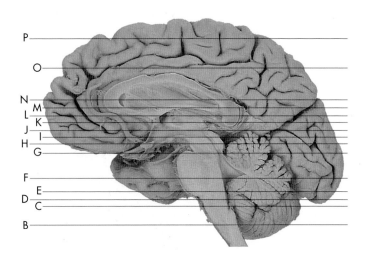

A, The planes of the "slices" shown in **B-P.**

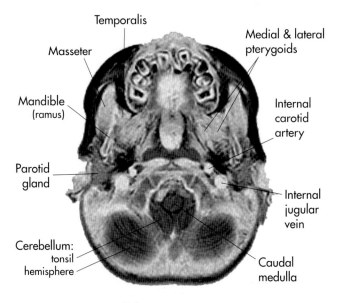

Temporalis

Masseter

Medial & lateral pterygoids

Mandible (ramus)

Internal carotid artery

Parotid gland

Internal jugular vein

Cerebellum: tonsil hemisphere

Caudal medulla

B, Foramen magnum.

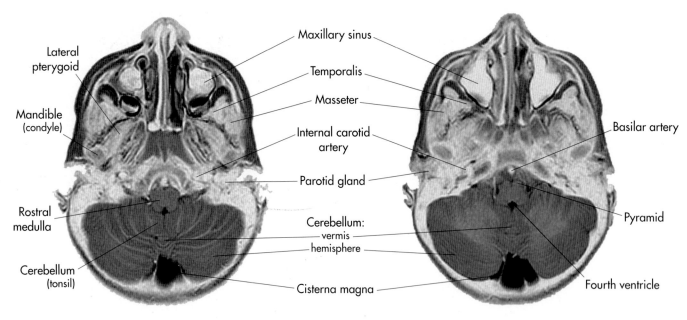

Lateral pterygoid

Mandible (condyle)

Rostral medulla

Cerebellum (tonsil)

Maxillary sinus

Temporalis

Masseter

Internal carotid artery

Parotid gland

Cerebellum: vermis hemisphere

Cisterna magna

Basilar artery

Pyramid

Fourth ventricle

C, Rostral medulla.   **D,** Rostral medulla.

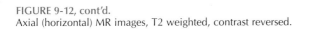

FIGURE 9-12, cont'd.
Axial (horizontal) MR images, T2 weighted, contrast reversed.

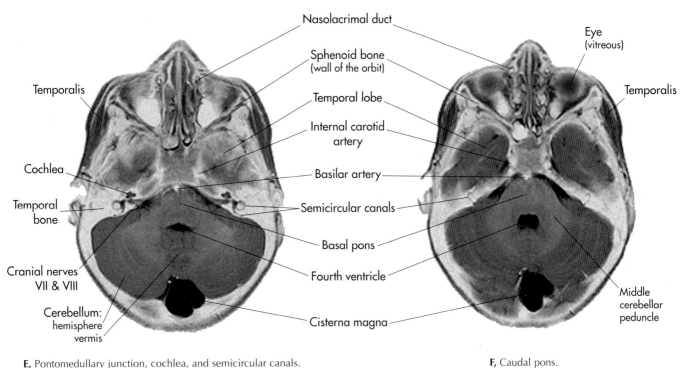

E, Pontomedullary junction, cochlea, and semicircular canals.

F, Caudal pons.

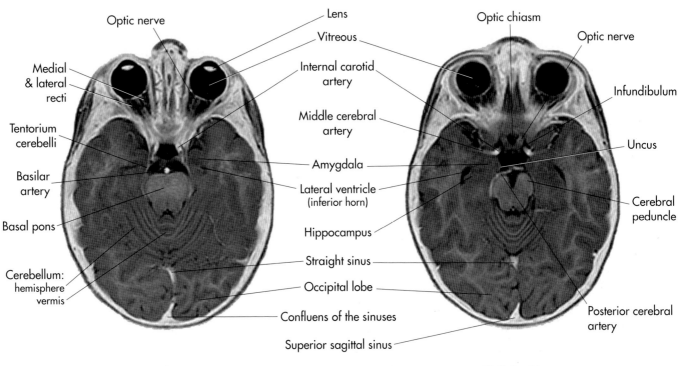

G, Rostral pons.

H, Optic chiasm.

FIGURE 9-12, cont'd.
Axial (horizontal) MR images, T2 weighted, contrast reversed.

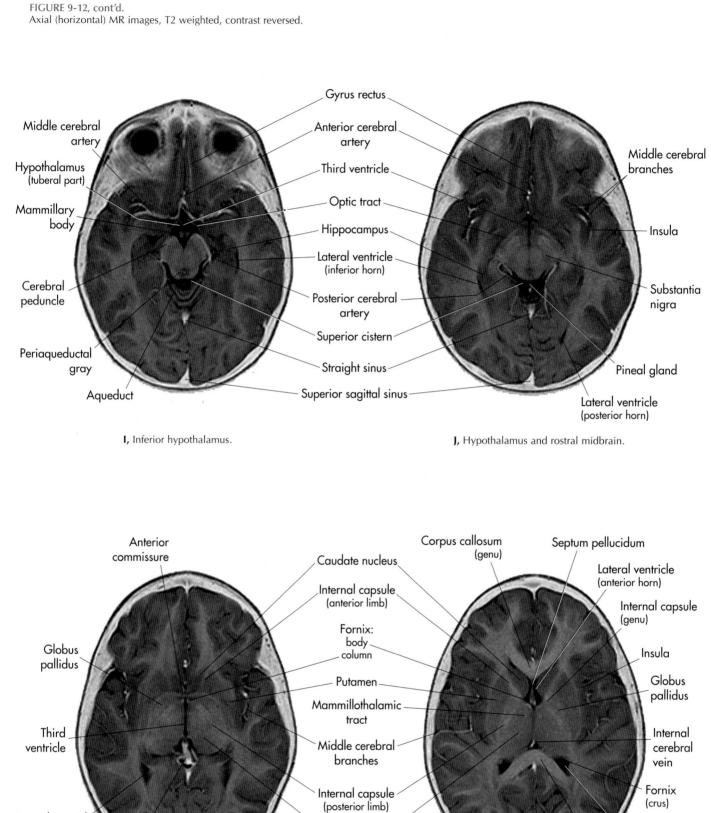

Middle cerebral artery

Hypothalamus (tuberal part)

Mammillary body

Cerebral peduncle

Periaqueductal gray

Aqueduct

Gyrus rectus

Anterior cerebral artery

Third ventricle

Optic tract

Hippocampus

Lateral ventricle (inferior horn)

Posterior cerebral artery

Superior cistern

Straight sinus

Superior sagittal sinus

Middle cerebral branches

Insula

Substantia nigra

Pineal gland

Lateral ventricle (posterior horn)

I, Inferior hypothalamus.

J, Hypothalamus and rostral midbrain.

Anterior commissure

Globus pallidus

Third ventricle

Lateral ventricle (inferior horn)

Great cerebral vein (of Galen)

Caudate nucleus

Internal capsule (anterior limb)

Fornix: body column

Putamen

Mammillothalamic tract

Middle cerebral branches

Internal capsule (posterior limb)

Thalamus

Superior sagittal sinus

Corpus callosum (genu)

Septum pellucidum

Lateral ventricle (anterior horn)

Internal capsule (genu)

Insula

Globus pallidus

Internal cerebral vein

Fornix (crus)

Lateral ventricle (atrium)

Corpus callosum (splenium)

Posterior cerebral branches

K, Anterior commissure.

L, Genu and splenium of the corpus callosum.

FIGURE 9-12, cont'd.
Axial (horizontal) MR images, T2 weighted, contrast reversed.

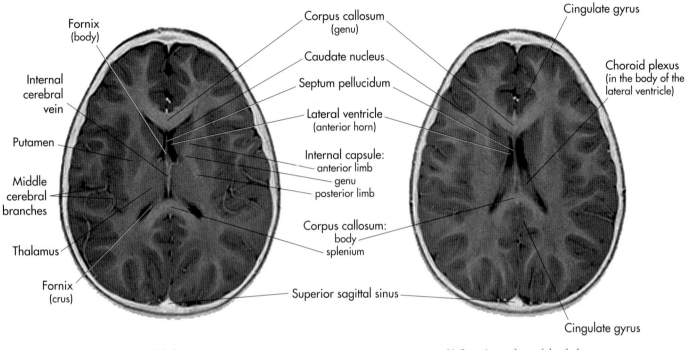

Fornix (body)

Internal cerebral vein

Putamen

Middle cerebral branches

Thalamus

Fornix (crus)

Corpus callosum (genu)

Caudate nucleus

Septum pellucidum

Lateral ventricle (anterior horn)

Internal capsule:
anterior limb
genu
posterior limb

Corpus callosum:
body
splenium

Superior sagittal sinus

Cingulate gyrus

Choroid plexus (in the body of the lateral ventricle)

Cingulate gyrus

M, Midthalamus.

N, Superior surface of the thalamus.

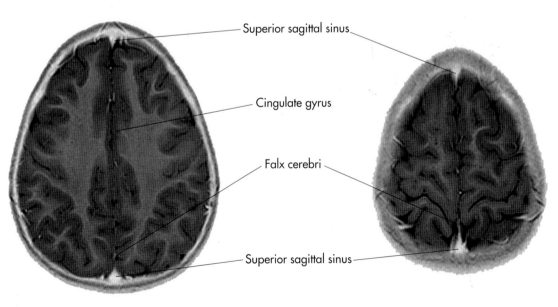

Superior sagittal sinus

Cingulate gyrus

Falx cerebri

Superior sagittal sinus

O, Just above the corpus callosum.

P, Near the top of the head.

FIGURE 9-13
Sagittal and parasagittal MR images, T2 weighted, contrast reversed.

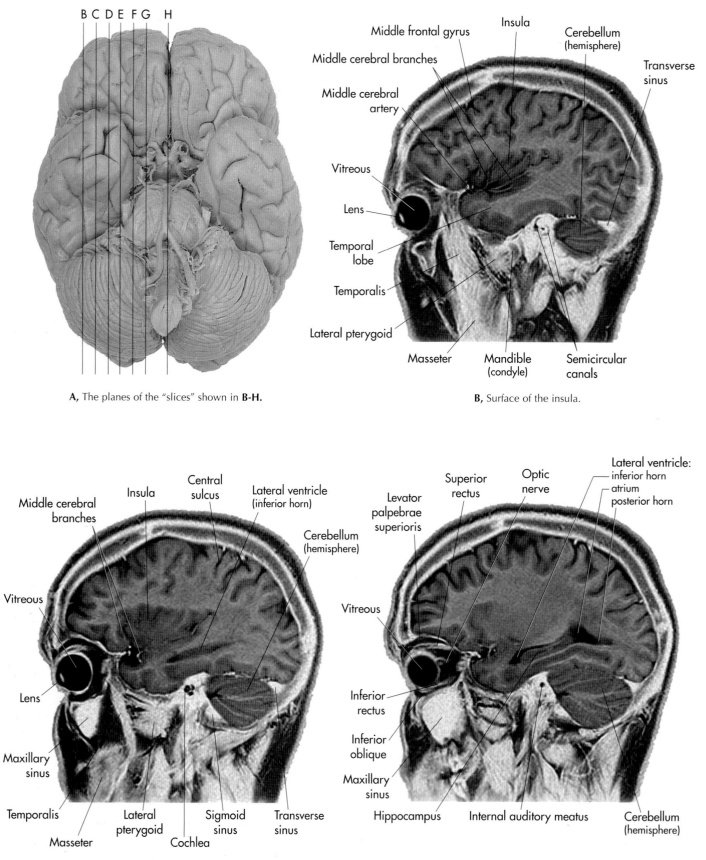

A, The planes of the "slices" shown in **B-H.**

B, Surface of the insula.

C, Inferior horn of the lateral ventricle.

D, Hippocampus.

FIGURE 9-13, cont'd.
Sagittal and parasagittal MR images, T2 weighted, contrast reversed.

E, Lenticular nucleus and thalamus.

F, Internal capsule.

G, Head of the caudate nucleus.

H, Near the midline.

FIGURE 9-14
The use of MR imaging to demonstrate intracranial pathology.

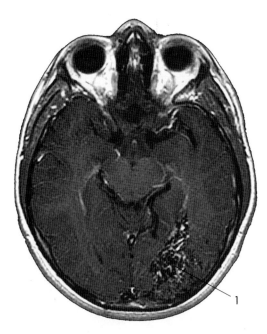

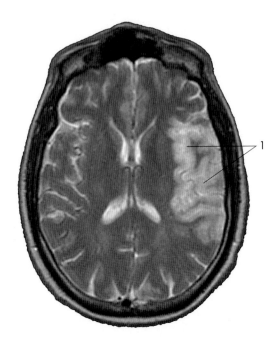

A, This T1-weighted image shows an arteriovenous malformation *(1)* in the occipital and temporal lobes. A contrast agent (gadolinium) effective in MR studies was injected intravenously before the study, so some of the vessels look brighter than would be expected otherwise.

B, This T2-weighted image demonstrates the results of a stroke in the territory of the left middle cerebral artery. The damaged cerebral cortex *(1)* is edematous and the increased water concentration makes it appear lighter than neighboring cortex.

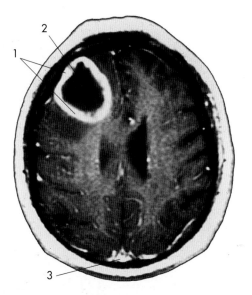

C, A T1-weighted image of a patient with an abscess in the right frontal lobe. Gadolinium was injected before the study, so some vessels (e.g., the superior sagittal sinus, *3*) can be seen. In addition, the abscess is revealed to have two parts: a rim of damaged tissue *(1)*, with a disrupted blood-brain barrier that allowed the contrast agent to leak out, and a fluid-filled necrotic core *(2)*.

D, A T1-weighted image of a patient with a tumor (*3*, a glioblastoma multiforme) in the left occipital and parietal lobes. The tumor has a disrupted blood-brain barrier that allows contrast material to leak into it, and adjacent areas *(2)* appear darker than normal because of edema. The tumor has compressed the left lateral ventricle *(1)* and shifted parts of the left hemisphere to the right.

Blood vessels can be visualized with most imaging techniques by finding a way to make the blood contained within them differ in some way from surrounding structures. Cerebral angiography utilizes the intravenous injection of iodinated dyes to make blood much more opaque than brain to x-rays (Figure 9-15). More recently, MR imaging techniques that depend on the intrinsic properties of flowing blood have been developed (Figure 9-16). MR angiography has the advantage of being completely noninvasive—no intravenous contrast material is required—but the resulting images are not as detailed as those produced by traditional angiography.

A cerebral angiogram is typically produced by introducing a catheter into the femoral artery, threading it (under fluoroscopic control) up the aorta and into the aortic arch, then steering the catheter tip into the artery of interest. In this way, the contrast material can be introduced into a single vertebral or internal carotid artery. Once the dye has been introduced, a rapid series of radiographs can follow it as it flows through the artery, into capillaries, and then into veins (Figure 9-15). Finally, photographic* (as in Figure 9-15) or digital (Figure 9-21, A and B) techniques can be used to remove bone images and reveal blood vessels in relative isolation.

*A radiographic image is made before injection of the iodinated dye and its contrast is reversed (i.e., a positive image is made, so that bone is dark). The reverse-contrast image is stacked on top of the image made after dye injection and a print made of both together. The reciprocally contrasting portions of the two images thus provide a relatively uniform background from which the blood vessels stand out.

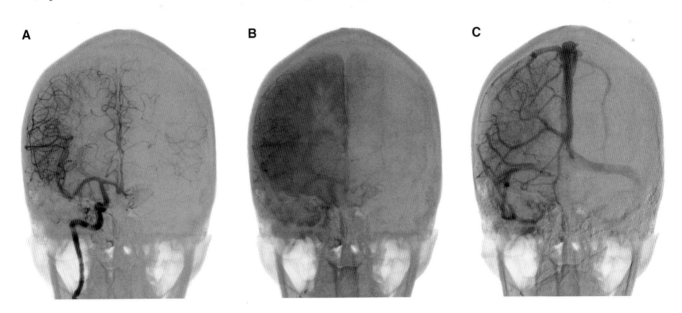

A **B** **C**

FIGURE 9-15
Movement of contrast material through the intracranial vasculature, as seen in a series of anteroposterior (AP) views (as though you are looking at the patient's forehead) after injection of the right internal carotid artery. **A,** About 2 seconds after injection, the arteries are filled. **B,** About 5 seconds after injection, the contrast has moved out of arteries and into capillary beds. **C,** About 7 seconds after injection, the contrast agent has moved into veins and venous sinuses.

FIGURE 9-16
MR angiography uses some of the intrinsic properties of flowing blood to create images of parts of the vasculature; appropriate adjustments of technical parameters can emphasize arteries or veins. The views in these images are as though you were looking up from below *(right)* or from the front *(below)* at the entire arterial supply of the brain. The internal carotid artery can be seen ascending through the neck *(11),* traversing the temporal bone *(3),* and passing through the cavernous sinus *(2).* The other arteries of the circle of Willis can also been seen—the anterior cerebral *(1),* posterior cerebral *(4),* and anterior *(13)* and posterior *(7)* communicating arteries—in addition to the middle cerebral artery *(9),* its branches on the surface of the insula *(8),* the vertebral *(12)* and basilar *(5)* arteries, the superior sagittal sinus *(6),* and even the ophthalmic artery *(10).*

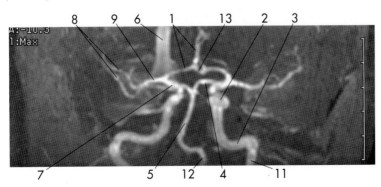

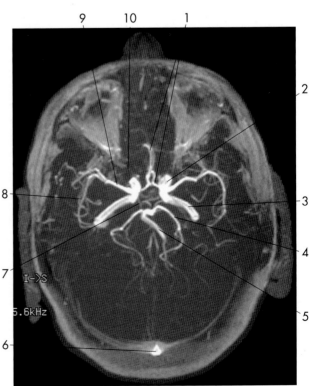

FIGURE 9-17
The arterial phase of a right internal carotid angiogram. **A,** A lateral view; the patient's face is to the right. **B,** An AP projection; the view is as though you were looking at the patient's forehead.

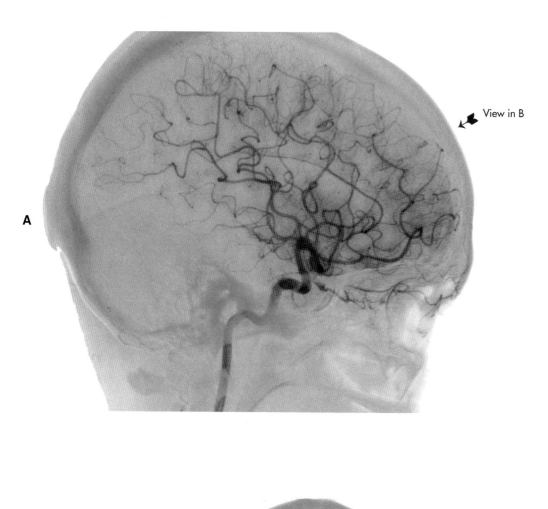

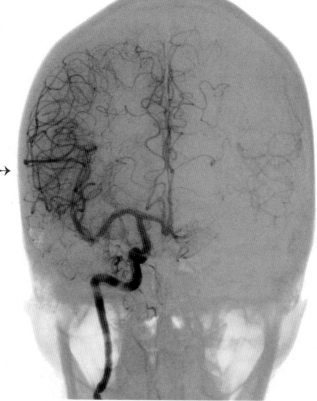

FIGURE 9-17, cont'd.
C, The internal carotid artery bifurcates into the anterior and middle cerebral arteries. The anterior cerebral artery in turn gives rise to two prominent branches, the pericallosal (➤) and callosomarginal (➤) arteries, which curve around above the corpus callosum and supply most of the medial surface of the cerebral hemisphere. Branches of the middle cerebral artery traverse the insula (➤), emerge from the lateral sulcus (☞), and supply the lateral surface of the hemisphere. **D,** In an AP projection the separation between anterior and middle cerebral territories can be seen more easily.

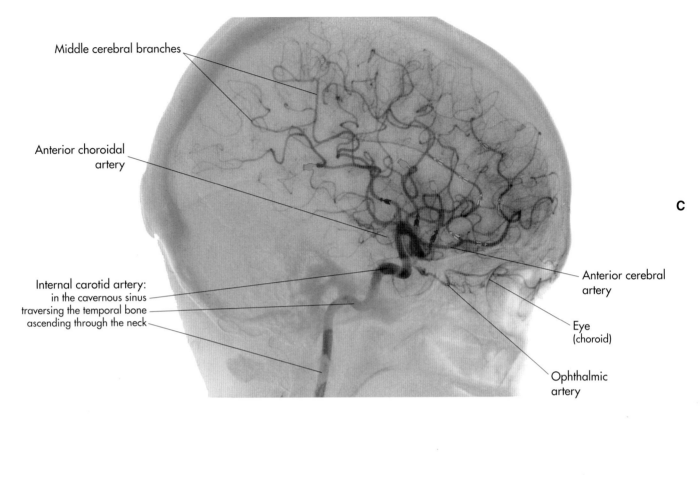

FIGURE 9-18
The venous phase of a right internal carotid angiogram. **A,** A lateral view; the patient's face is to the right. **B,** An AP projection; the view is as though you were looking at the patient's forehead. Flow into the transverse sinuses is typically asymmetrical; in this patient most blood from the superior sagittal sinus flows into the left transverse sinus (more commonly it flows to the right).

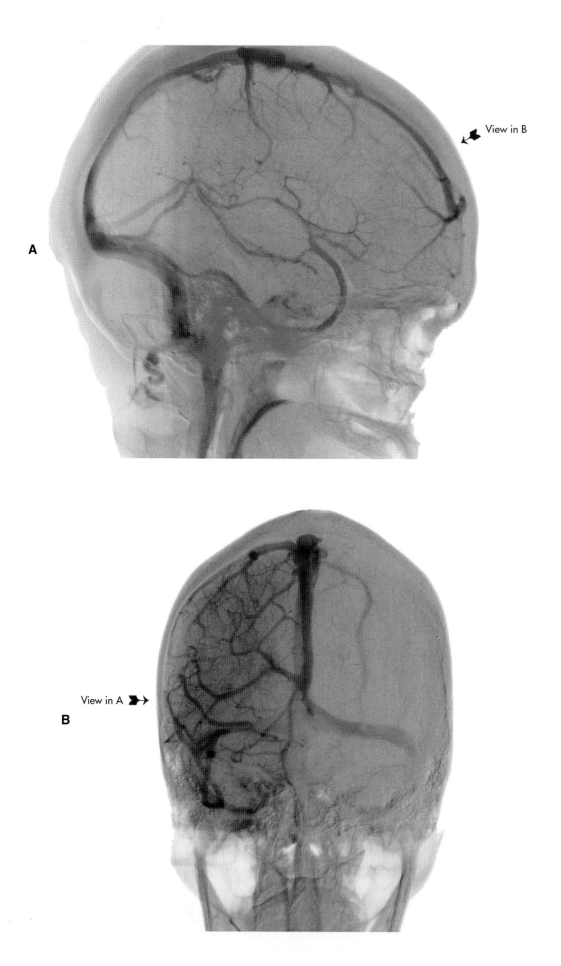

FIGURE 9-18, cont'd.
C, Blood flows through a system of deep veins (➤➤) to the straight and transverse sinuses and through a system of superficial veins (➤➤) to the superior sagittal sinus; both systems meet at the confluens of the sinuses. **D,** In an AP view, the superior sagittal sinus occupies much of the midline, obscuring other vessels.

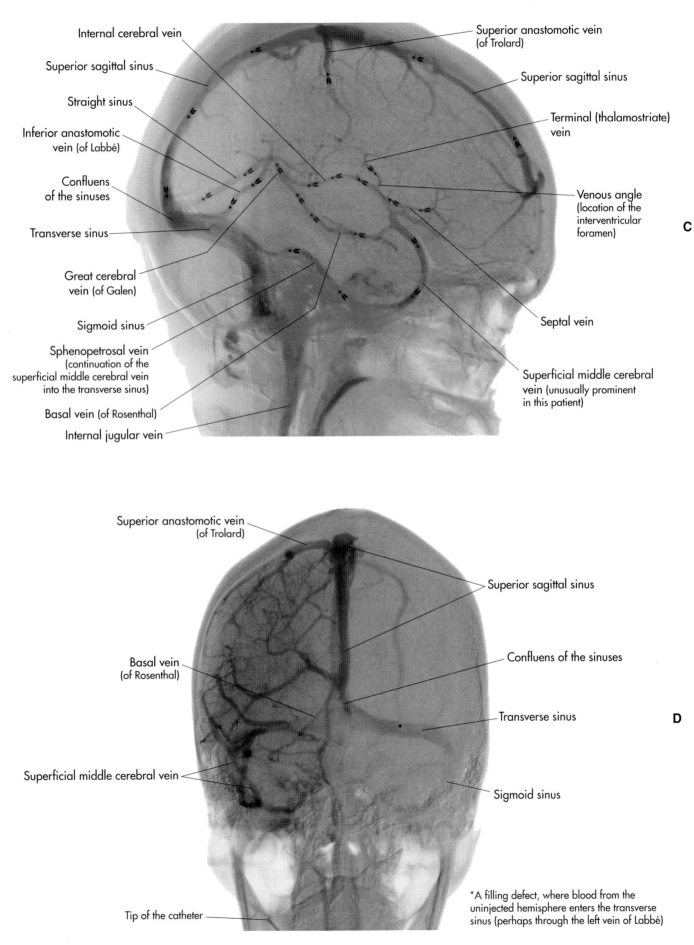

Internal cerebral vein

Superior sagittal sinus

Straight sinus

Inferior anastomotic
vein (of Labbé)

Confluens
of the sinuses

Transverse sinus

Great cerebral
vein (of Galen)

Sigmoid sinus

Sphenopetrosal vein
(continuation of the
superficial middle cerebral vein
into the transverse sinus)

Basal vein (of Rosenthal)

Internal jugular vein

Superior anastomotic vein
(of Trolard)

Superior sagittal sinus

Terminal (thalamostriate)
vein

Venous angle
(location of the
interventricular
foramen)

Septal vein

Superficial middle cerebral
vein (unusually prominent
in this patient)

C

Superior anastomotic vein
(of Trolard)

Basal vein
(of Rosenthal)

Superficial middle cerebral vein

Tip of the catheter

Superior sagittal sinus

Confluens of the sinuses

Transverse sinus

Sigmoid sinus

D

*A filling defect, where blood from the
uninjected hemisphere enters the transverse
sinus (perhaps through the left vein of Labbé)

FIGURE 9-19
The arterial phase of a left vertebral-basilar angiogram. **A,** A lateral view; the patient's face is to the right. **B,** An AP projection; the view is as though you were looking at the patient's forehead. In **B,** the basilar artery appears shorter than it really is because of the angle of view—you are looking almost longitudinally along it. (The right vertebral artery is visible because the pressure of the injection propelled some contrast material into it.)

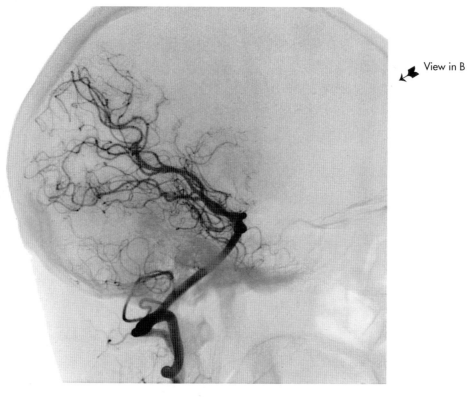

A

View in B

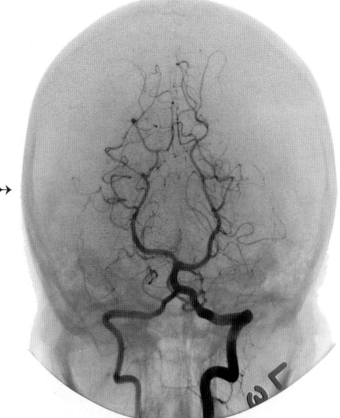

View in A

B

FIGURE 9-19, cont'd.
C, The vertebral and basilar arteries and their branches supply areas below the tentorium cerebelli (location indicated by *), and the posterior cerebral arteries supply parts of the midbrain and supratentorial structures (including much of the thalamus). **D,** the two vertebral arteries (➤➤) join to form a single, midline basilar artery (➤➤), which gives rise to a series of branches as it courses along the anterior surface of the pons, finally bifurcating at the level of the midbrain to form the two posterior cerebral arteries (➤➤).

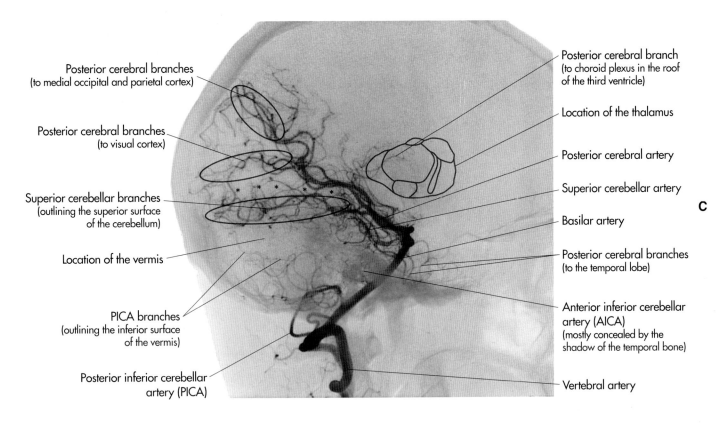

Posterior cerebral branches
(to medial occipital and parietal cortex)

Posterior cerebral branches
(to visual cortex)

Superior cerebellar branches
(outlining the superior surface
of the cerebellum)

Location of the vermis

PICA branches
(outlining the inferior surface
of the vermis)

Posterior inferior cerebellar
artery (PICA)

Posterior cerebral branch
(to choroid plexus in the roof
of the third ventricle)

Location of the thalamus

Posterior cerebral artery

Superior cerebellar artery

Basilar artery

Posterior cerebral branches
(to the temporal lobe)

Anterior inferior cerebellar
artery (AICA)
(mostly concealed by the
shadow of the temporal bone)

Vertebral artery

C

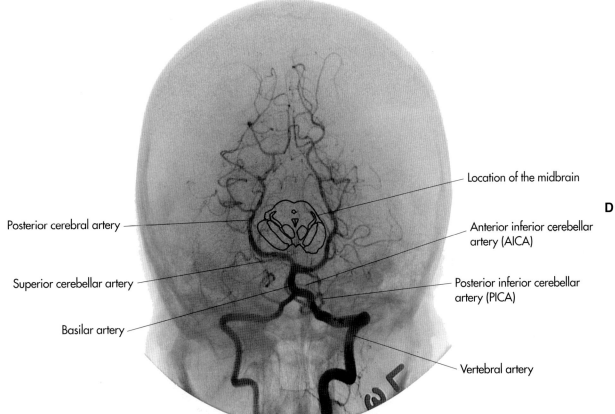

Posterior cerebral artery

Superior cerebellar artery

Basilar artery

Location of the midbrain

Anterior inferior cerebellar
artery (AICA)

Posterior inferior cerebellar
artery (PICA)

Vertebral artery

D

FIGURE 9-20

The venous phase of a vertebral angiogram. **A,** A lateral view; the patient's face is to the right. **B,** An AP projection; the view is as though you were looking at the patient's forehead. Flow into the transverse sinuses is typically asymmetrical; in this patient most blood from the superior sagittal sinus appears to flow into the left transverse sinus.

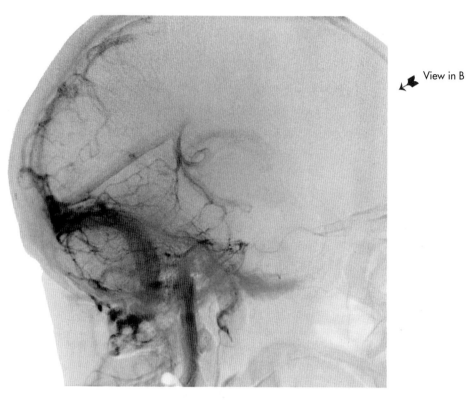

A

View in B

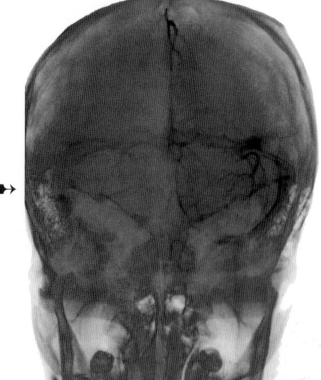

B   View in A

FIGURE 9-20, cont'd.
C, A network of veins drains from the cerebellum and brainstem into the great vein or straight sinus (➤➤), or into the transverse or petrosal sinuses. The medial surface of the occipital lobe drains into the superior sagittal sinus (➤➤). **D,** In an AP view, the straight sinus is seen almost end-on.

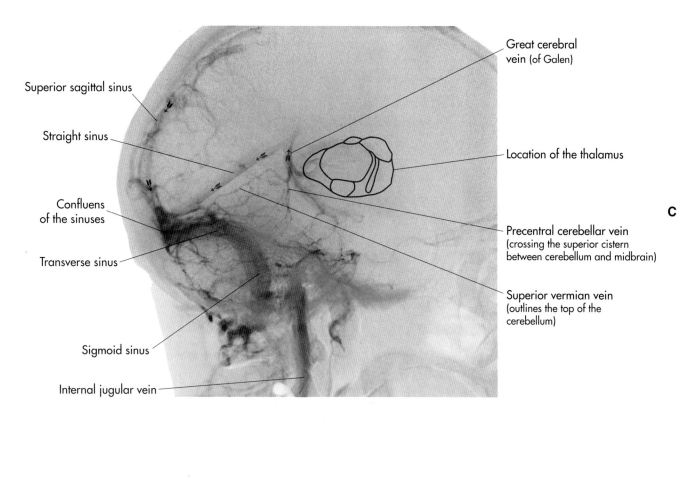

Superior sagittal sinus

Straight sinus

Confluens
of the sinuses

Transverse sinus

Sigmoid sinus

Internal jugular vein

Great cerebral
vein (of Galen)

Location of the thalamus

Precentral cerebellar vein
(crossing the superior cistern
between cerebellum and midbrain)

Superior vermian vein
(outlines the top of the
cerebellum)

C

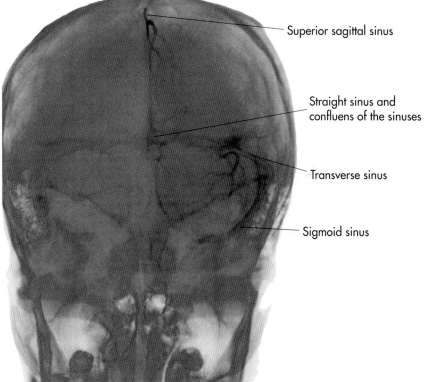

Superior sagittal sinus

Straight sinus and
confluens of the sinuses

Transverse sinus

Sigmoid sinus

D

FIGURE 9-21
The use of angiography to demonstrate intracranial pathology.

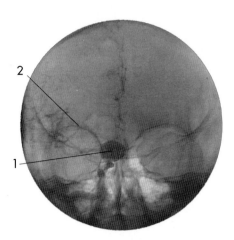

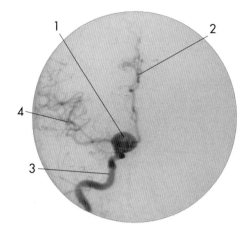

A, In this AP view, an aneurysm (a balloon-like swelling of the wall of an artery) can be seen *(1)*, but the x-ray density of bony structures such as those around the orbit *(2)* obscures many details.

B, The same patient as in **A;** digital processing has removed the bony structures. The aneurysm *(1)*, arising at the origin of the ophthalmic artery, can be seen more clearly, as can the internal carotid artery *(3)* and branches of the anterior *(2)* and middle *(4)* cerebral arteries.

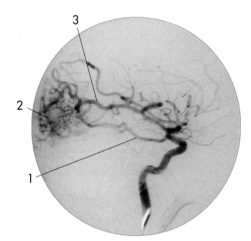

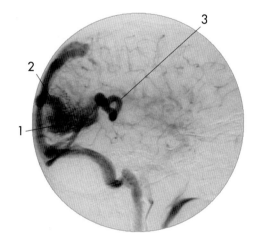

C, An arteriovenous malformation *(2)* in the occipital lobe, fed by enlarged branches of the middle *(3)* and posterior *(1)* cerebral arteries. This patient's posterior cerebral artery originates directly from the internal carotid—a common variant. Lateral view, anterior to the right.

D, The same arteriovenous malformation *(1)* shown in **C,** draining through distended venous channels *(2, 3)* into the straight and superior sagittal sinuses.

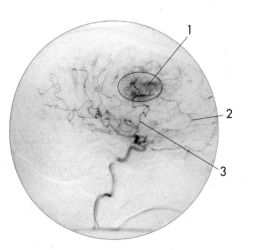

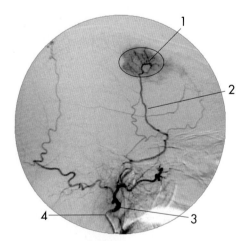

E, A meningioma *(1)* growing from the falx cerebri. The tumor receives part of its blood supply from a branch *(3)* of the middle cerebral artery and possibly from a branch of the anterior cerebral artery *(2)*. Lateral view, anterior to the right.

F, The same meningioma *(1)* as in **E,** now seen after contrast was injected into the external carotid artery *(3;* note the catheter tip at *4)*. The tumor also gets some of its arterial supply from an abnormally large middle meningeal artery *(2)*.

This chapter provides brief descriptions and definitions of the neuroanatomical structures labeled in the preceding chapters. (The bones and muscles indicated in Chapter 9 are not defined, however.) Additional details can be found in standard neuroscience texts.

Although all of these definitions were written specifically for this atlas, many are adapted from passages in Nolte's *The Human Brain,* fourth edition.* Some others derive, with modifications, from a text by Jay Angevine (with Carl W. Cotman), *Principles of Neuroanatomy.*† We thank Jeffrey House of Oxford University Press for permission to draw upon the latter source.

Abducens nerve. The 6th cranial nerve, which emerges anteriorly from the brainstem between the pons and medulla. It innervates the lateral rectus muscle of the ipsilateral eye, affecting abduction (hence its name).

Abducens nucleus. Contains the lower motor neurons for the ipsilateral lateral rectus muscle, as well as interneurons that project through the contralateral MLF to medial rectus motor neurons; this feature provides for conjugate horizontal eye movements.

Accessory nerve. The 11th cranial nerve, which emerges laterally from the upper cervical cord and innervates the sternocleidomastoid and trapezius muscles to mediate turning the head and elevating the shoulder. (The accessory nerve is sometimes considered to have both cranial and spinal parts. The spinal part corresponds to the accessory nerve as defined here, and the cranial part to a series of rootlets that emerge laterally from the caudal medulla, join the vagus, and run to the palate, pharynx, and larynx with the vagus nerve.)

Ambient cistern. The combination of the superior cistern and sheetlike extensions from it that partially encircle the midbrain.

Amygdala. A collection of nuclei in the anteromedial part of the temporal lobe, just beneath the uncus, forming the core of one of the two major limbic circuits. (The core of the other is the hippocampus.)

Angular gyrus. That part of the inferior parietal lobule formed by the cortex surrounding the upturned end of the superior temporal sulcus; although variable in size and shape, this region is important in language function.

Ansa lenticularis. Part of the projection from the globus pallidus to the thalamus. It has fewer axons than the other part (see *lenticular fasciculus*). It forms a compact, conspicuous cable of myelinated fibers running beneath the internal capsule and hooking around its medial edge.

Anterior cerebral artery. The more anterior of the two terminal branches of the internal carotid artery. It curves around the corpus callosum with branches supplying orbital cortex, the medial surface of the frontal and parietal lobes, and an adjoining narrow band of cortex along their superior surfaces.

Anterior choroidal artery. A long, thin, branch of the internal carotid artery that accompanies the optic tract and supplies many structures along the way: the optic tract, choroid plexus of the inferior horn of the lateral ventricle, part of the cerebral peduncle, and deep regions of the internal capsule, thalamus, and hippocampus.

Anterior commissure. A small, sharply defined bundle of commissural fibers just beneath and behind the rostrum of the corpus callosum, to which it is closely related developmentally; a few inconspicuous anterior fibers interconnect olfactory structures, whereas its many large posterior fibers link the temporal cortex of the two sides of the brain.

Anterior communicating artery. A short vessel at the anterior end of the circle of Willis interconnecting the two anterior cerebral arteries just anterior to the optic chiasm; occasionally it may be very small or, very rarely, absent.

Anterior corticospinal tract. The smaller of the two corticospinal tracts. It consists of the fibers (about 15%) in each medullary pyramid that continue directly into the anterior funiculus of the spinal cord without decussating; many fibers eventually cross in the anterior white commissure of the cord before terminating, but some end ipsilaterally. Fibers of the anterior corticospinal tract end (mainly in the cervical and thoracic spinal cord) on spinal motor neurons or nearby interneurons.

Anterior funiculus. One of the three major divisions of the spinal white matter (*funiculus* is Latin for "string" or "cord," as in the old term *funicular* for cable-car), the others being the lateral and posterior funiculi. The anterior funiculus is located between the anterior median fissure and the exiting ventral roots and contains various tracts (mostly descending), including the anterior corticospinal tract.

Anterior horn. One of the three general divisions of the spinal gray matter, the others being the posterior horn and the intermediate zone; contains numerous local-circuit neurons, cell bodies of alpha (lower) motor neurons, axons of which enter the ventral (anterior) spinal nerve roots and end on skeletal muscle, and cell bodies of gamma motor neurons that regulate muscle spindles.

Anterior inferior cerebellar artery. A long, circumferential branch of the basilar artery arising just above the union of the two vertebrals. It supplies anterior regions of the inferior cerebellar surface, including the flocculus, and parts of the caudal pons; often referred to by the acronym AICA.

Anterior nucleus. See *thalamus.*

Anterior perforated substance. The inferior surface of the forebrain, roughly between the orbital gyri and the hypothalamus. So named because numerous lenticulostriate and other small ganglionic branches penetrate the brain here.

Anterior spinal artery. A single midline vessel that originates rostrally as two arteries (one from each vertebral), which shortly join and then course within the anterior median fissure along the entire spinal cord. It receives additional blood from the thoracic/abdominal aorta through numerous anastomoses with radicular arteries below the upper cervical region and gives rise to

*Nolte J: *The human brain,* ed 4, St. Louis, 1999, Mosby.
†Angevine JB Jr, Cotman CW: *Principles of neuroanatomy,* New York, 1981, Oxford University Press.

hundreds of central and circumferential branches that supply the anterior two thirds of the cord.

Anterior spinocerebellar tract. Crossed fibers from lumbosacral spinal gray matter, carrying mechanoreceptive and other information related to leg movement. The anterior spinocerebellar tract stays in a lateral position along the spinal cord and brainstem until the rostral pons, and there moves over the superior cerebellar peduncle and enters the cerebellum, where it largely recrosses.

Anterolateral system. An umbrella term for the spinothalamic tract and closely related ascending fibers, all of which deal with pain, temperature, and to some extent tactile/pressure sensation but many of which do not reach the thalamus, ending instead at higher spinal levels and/or in brainstem sites such as the reticular formation.

Aqueduct (of Sylvius). The narrow channel (a remnant of the lumen of the embryonic mesencephalon) through the midbrain connecting the third and fourth ventricles. The aqueduct lacks a choroid plexus and serves only as a conduit for cerebrospinal fluid descending through the ventricular system (its stenosis or obstruction is the most common cause of congenital hydrocephalus).

Arachnoid granulations. Small evaginations of the arachnoid membrane protruding through a hiatus in dural connective tissue into the lumen of a dural sinus of the brain (especially the superior sagittal sinus), so that only loosely arranged arachnoid cells and endothelium intervene between subarachnoid space and venous blood. Arachnoid granulations are the major (but not exclusive) sites of reabsorption of cerebrospinal fluid into the venous system.

Area postrema. A small region at the caudal end of the fourth ventricle where the ventricular walls join at the obex. The area postrema is one of several circumventricular organs of the brain where cerebral capillaries are fenestrated and allow free communication between the blood and brain extracellular fluid ("holes" in the blood-brain barrier); it is thought to monitor blood for toxins and to trigger vomiting.

Basal forebrain. A loosely used umbrella term for an area at and near the inferior surface of the telencephalon between the hypothalamus and orbital cortex. It includes the anterior perforated substance superficially and extends superiorly into the septal area and adjacent oxymoronically named *substantia innominata* (see also *basal nucleus*).

Basal nucleus (of Meynert). Groups of large cholinergic neurons in the substantia innominata of the basal forebrain. Widespread projections of these and nearby septal neurons blanket the neocortex, hippocampus, and amygdala with cholinergic endings, suggestive of general regulation of forebrain activity.

Basal pons. A mass of gray and white matter, transversely situated and filled with transversely and longitudinally coursing fibers, on the anterior surface of the pons. The basal pons looks like a bridge (for which the pons was named) between the two cerebellar hemispheres, but in fact it is a key link between the cerebrum and cerebellum: corticopontine fibers end in its scat-

tered pontine nuclei, which in turn project across the midline into the cerebellum via the middle cerebellar peduncle.

Basal vein (of Rosenthal). A deep cerebral vein whose tributaries drain the insula and some structures near the inferior surface of the forebrain. The basal vein then curves around the midbrain and joins the great cerebral vein.

Basilar artery. A large vessel formed by union of the two vertebral arteries. The basilar artery runs upward along the anterior median surface of the pons and gives rise to many branches that supply the pons, superior surface of the cerebellum, and caudal midbrain; it bifurcates at the level of the midbrain into the two posterior cerebral arteries.

Brachium of the inferior colliculus. Auditory afferents from the inferior colliculus on their way to the medial geniculate nucleus.

Brachium of the superior colliculus. A bundle of fibers that passes over the medial geniculate nucleus to reach the superior colliculus. Contains afferents from the retina that bypass the lateral geniculate nucleus and project directly to the superior colliculus and pretectal area, as well as projections from cerebral cortex to the superior colliculus.

Brainstem. In common medical usage, the midbrain, pons, and medulla. (Earlier definitions frequently included various parts of the diencephalon and telencephalon as well [e.g., thalamus, basal ganglia].)

Calcarine sulcus. A prominent, deep cerebral infolding. It originates anteriorly in the temporal lobe near the splenium of the corpus callosum and continues posteriorly into the occipital lobe, where it terminates at the occipital pole. Its upper and lower banks contain the primary visual cortex. Anteriorly along this course, the parietooccipital sulcus branches off from it.

Callosomarginal artery. A branch of the anterior cerebral artery that follows the cingulate sulcus.

Caudate nucleus. The more medial part of the striatum, bulging into the lateral ventricle with its large head in the wall of the anterior horn, tapering body immediately behind, and long slender tail running posteriorly into the atrium and then anteriorly into the inferior horn. It is principally connected with prefrontal and other association areas of cortex, and is involved more in cognitive functions and less directly in movement.

Central canal. The narrow, functionless vestige of the lumen of the spinal part of the embryonic neural tube, lined by ependyma and usually obstructed by epithelial debris. It runs the length of the spinal cord, contains traces of cerebrospinal fluid, and opens into the fourth ventricle at the obex of the medulla.

Central sulcus (of Rolando). An anatomically and functionally important infolding of the cerebral hemisphere, beginning just medial to its superior border, proceeding over its superior margin, and descending obliquely forward almost to the lateral sulcus. The central sulcus is the boundary between frontal and parietal lobes, and the transition zone between primary motor and primary somatosensory cortex.

Central tegmental tract. A complex, heterogeneous tract running centrally through each side of the brainstem reticular formation and providing a major highway through which reticular afferents and efferents are distributed. It also contains a major projection from the red nucleus to the inferior olivary nucleus, axons intrinsic to the reticular formation, and undoubtedly other types of fibers that are incompletely charted and understood.

Centromedian nucleus. See *thalamus.*

Cerebellothalamic tract. Efferent fibers from the deep cerebellar nuclei (mainly the dentate nucleus) passing via the superior cerebellar peduncle and its decussation through or around the contralateral red nucleus to the ventral lateral nucleus of the thalamus for projection to motor areas of cortex. This tract completes a long, doubly-crossed circuit between each cerebral hemisphere and the contralateral cerebellar hemisphere that is crucial for the planning and coordination of skilled volitional movement. Because most of its fibers arise in the dentate nucleus, the cerebellothalamic tract is sometimes referred to as the *dentatothalamic tract.*

Cerebellum. A large, convoluted subdivision of the nervous system (cerebellum literally means "little brain") that receives input from sensory systems, the cerebral cortex, and other sites and participates in the planning and coordination of movement.
Anterior lobe. All of the cerebellum anterior to the primary fissure (partly vermis, partly hemisphere).
Flocculus. The hemispheral component of the flocculonodular lobe, the part of the cerebellum particularly concerned with the vestibular system and eye movements.
Hemispheres. The large paired lateral parts, important for coordination of the limbs.
Nodulus. The vermal component of the flocculonodular lobe, the part of the cerebellum particularly concerned with the vestibular system and eye movements.
Posterior lobe. All of the cerebellum, except for the flocculonodular lobe, posterior to the primary fissure (partly vermis, partly hemisphere).
Primary fissure. Separates the anterior and posterior lobes of the cerebellum.
Tonsil. A medial, inferior part of the posterior lobe hemisphere, adjacent to the medulla as it passes through the foramen magnum. (See Figure 9-6, *B.*)
Vermis. (Latin for "worm"), the most medial zone of the cerebellum, straddling the midline.

Cerebral peduncle. As the term is used in this book, a massive sheaf of tightly packed corticospinal, corticobulbar, and corticopontine fibers traveling along the base of the midbrain. (Others use the term *cerebral peduncle* to refer to all of one side of the midbrain inferior to the aqueduct. In this terminology, the bundle of corticofugal fibers is called the *pes pedunculi, basis pedunculi,* or *crus cerebri.*)

Choroid plexus. Long, grapevinelike, highly convoluted, vascularized strands in the lateral, third, and fourth ventricles in which most of the cerebrospinal fluid is produced.
Glomus. An enlarged strand of choroid plexus in the atrium of the lateral ventricle. The glomus accumulates calcium deposits with age, and so can often be seen in CT images.

Choroid fissure. A C-shaped fissure on the medial surface of each cerebral hemisphere, leading into the choroid plexus of the lateral ventricle.

Choroidal vein. A tortuous vessel entering the terminal (thalamostriate) vein near the interventricular foramen and draining the choroid plexus of the body of the lateral ventricle.

Cingulate gyrus. A broad belt of cortex partially encircling the corpus callosum. The cingulate gyrus forms the upper part of the limbic lobe (see *parahippocampal gyrus*) and has extensive limbic connections, particularly in cortical circuits leading ultimately to or from the hippocampus.

Cingulate sulcus. A more or less continuous, curved infolding of each cerebral hemisphere clearly demarcating the outer margin of the cingulate gyrus; posteriorly a branch (the marginal branch) ascends to the superior margin of the parietal lobe immediately behind the upper end of the central sulcus.

Cisterna magna. A large subarachnoid cistern between the medulla and the inferior vermis. Also referred to as the *cerebellomedullary cistern.*

Clarke's nucleus (nucleus dorsalis). A rounded group of large cell bodies in the intermediate spinal gray near the medial edge of the base of the posterior horn, from about T1 through L2 or L3. Clarke's nucleus is the origin of the posterior spinocerebellar tract, through which stretch receptor and other mechanoreceptive input from the leg reaches the ipsilateral cerebellar vermis and intermediate zone.

Claustrum. A thin but extensive layer of gray matter beneath the insula, separated from it and the underlying putamen by the extreme and external capsules, respectively. The claustrum has reciprocal connections with cerebral cortex, but incompletely understood functions.

Cochlear nuclei. The nuclei in which the primary auditory afferents of the cochlear nerve terminate. The dorsal and ventral cochlear nuclei form a continuous band of gray matter draped over the inferior cerebellar peduncle near the pontomedullary junction, and project bilaterally to the superior olivary nucleus and into the lateral lemniscus.

Collateral sulcus. A deep infolding of the inferior surface of the temporal lobe, bulging into the wall of the inferior horn of the lateral ventricle as the collateral eminence. It separates the occipitotemporal (fusiform) gyrus from the parahippocampal gyrus.

Corpus callosum. (Latin for "hard body"), a massive curvilinear bridge of commissural fibers, shaped in sagittal aspect like an overturned canoe. The corpus callosum interconnects most cortical areas of the two cerebral hemispheres and serves to join them functionally, providing the substrate for a unitary consciousness.
Body. The main arched part of the corpus callosum. Its fibers distribute extensively within each hemisphere.
Genu. The kneelike sharp anterior bend, containing fibers that lead to the frontal lobes.

Rostrum. The slender, narrow part beneath the genu, resembling the prow of the (overturned) boat; interconnects orbital cortex.

Splenium. The thick, rounded posterior bend (like a rolled bandage), containing fibers to occipital and temporal regions.

Corticobulbar tract. Strictly defined, a large collection of fibers originating in the cerebral cortex and descending through the internal capsule (immediately anterior to the closely related corticospinal fibers) to terminate (via numerous, often intricate routes) in the "bulb" (an old term for the medulla or, by extension, for the entire brainstem) on neurons of sensory relay nuclei, the reticular formation, and motor nuclei of cranial nerves. In common usage, the term refers only to the last fibers of this group. Basically, the equivalent of the corticospinal tract for cranial nerve nuclei.

Corticopontine tract. A very large collection of fibers originating in frontal, parietal, occipital, and temporal cortex and descending through the internal capsule (immediately anterior and posterior to the corticospinal/corticobulbar projections) to nuclei in the basal pons, from which axons pass to the contralateral cerebellar hemispheres through the middle cerebellar peduncles.

Corticospinal tract. A collection of about a million axons that originate in the cerebral cortex, descend through the internal capsule, cerebral peduncle, basal pons, and medullary pyramid, then reach the spinal cord, where they terminate, via the lateral and anterior corticospinal tracts. Roughly a third of them originate in primary motor cortex, the rest arising from premotor and supplementary motor areas and the parietal lobe (especially somatosensory cortex). Corticospinal axons end in the spinal cord on cells of the posterior horn, intermediate gray, and anterior horn, where some synapse directly on alpha and gamma motor neurons. A single functional role is difficult to specify, but this is the principal pathway for the production of skilled volitional movements.

Cuneate tubercle. A conspicuous swelling on the dorsolateral aspect of the lower medulla overlying the cuneate nucleus, which mediates that part of the posterior column–medial lemniscus pathway carrying tactile and proprioceptive information from the arm and upper body.

Cuneus. The wedge-shaped area of medial occipital cortex between the calcarine and parietooccipital sulci. Includes the upper half of primary visual cortex.

Dentate ligament. A thickened, lateral, serrated sheet of the pia mater on each side of the spinal cord, with periodic extensions that attach to the arachnoid and dura, stabilizing the position of the cord within the dural sac.

Dentate nucleus. The largest and most lateral of the deep cerebellar nuclei, featuring a highly convoluted narrow band of neurons arranged like a bag, with an anteriorly directed opening (hilus) from which efferents emerge to form most of the superior cerebellar peduncle.

Diencephalon. Literally the "betweenbrain," the caudal subdivision of the embryonic forebrain, giving rise to the pineal gland, habenula, thalamus, subthalamic nucleus, retina, optic nerve and tract, hypothalamus, infundibulum (pituitary stalk), and neurohypophysis.

Dorsal cochlear nucleus. See *cochlear nuclei.*

Dorsal longitudinal fasciculus. Ascending and descending fibers connecting the hypothalamus to the reticular formation and to preganglionic autonomic neurons, traveling through the periaqueductal and periventricular gray matter.

Dorsal motor nucleus of the vagus. A prominent autonomic efferent nucleus containing most of the preganglionic parasympathetic neurons for thoracic and abdominal viscera.

Dorsal root. The posterior, sensory root of a spinal nerve, which divides into a variable number of regularly spaced rootlets that enter the spinal cord along its posterolateral sulcus.

Dorsomedial nucleus. See *thalamus.*

Edinger-Westphal nucleus. A column of small nerve cell bodies near the midline of the oculomotor nucleus. Its neurons form the efferent arm of the direct and consensual pupillary light reflexes: preganglionic parasympathetic neurons affect (via postganglionic neurons in the ciliary ganglion) contraction of the pupillary sphincter to constrict the pupil. Also part of the efferent arm of the near reflex: it mediates (again via postganglionic neurons in the ciliary ganglion) ciliary muscle contraction to thicken the lens and pupillary constriction to increase depth of focus.

Entorhinal cortex. The cortex covering the anterior part of the parahippocampal gyrus, near the uncus. Entorhinal cortex receives inputs from the amygdala, olfactory bulb, the limbic lobe, and other cortical areas, and in turn is the major source of afferents to the hippocampus.

External medullary lamina (of the thalamus). A thin, curved sheet of myelinated fibers (afferent and efferent), in places fenestrated and in others dense, surrounding the lateral surface of the thalamus; enclosed by a thin shell of gray matter, the reticular nucleus (see *thalamus*), which intervenes between it and the internal capsule.

Facial colliculus. A swelling in the floor of the fourth ventricle, caused by the underlying internal genu of the facial nerve looping around the abducens nucleus.

Facial nerve. The 7th cranial nerve, which emerges anterolaterally from the brainstem along the groove between the basal pons and the medulla. The facial nerve serves nasopharyngeal, taste, and external ear sensation; controls muscles of facial expression; and regulates secretion by the submandibular, sublingual, and lacrimal glands.

Facial nucleus. A group of lower motor neurons that innervate muscles of the ipsilateral half of the face.

Fasciculus cuneatus. Uncrossed, large, myelinated, primary afferents entering the posterior column of the spinal cord rostral to T6 and carrying tactile and proprioceptive information from the arm; many of these fibers ascend to the medulla to terminate in nucleus cuneatus.

Fasciculus gracilis. Uncrossed, large, myelinated, primary afferents entering the posterior column of the spinal cord caudal to

T6 and carrying tactile and proprioceptive information from the leg; many of these fibers ascend to the medulla to terminate in nucleus gracilis.

Fastigial nucleus. The most medial of the deep cerebellar nuclei. Its afferents come mainly from the cerebellar vermis, and its efferents project bilaterally to the vestibular nuclei and reticular formation.

Fimbria. (Literally the "fringe"), a prominent band of white matter along the medial edge of the hippocampus. The fimbria is an accumulation of myelinated axons (mostly efferent) that first collect on the ventricular surface of the hippocampus as the alveus (a thin layer resembling an inverted trough). Near the splenium the fimbria separates from the hippocampus as the crus of the fornix.

Flocculus. The hemispheral component of the flocculonodular lobe, the part of the cerebellum particularly concerned with the vestibular system and eye movements.

Foramen of Monro. See *interventricular foramen.*

Fornix. A prominent paired fiber bundle, mostly containing hippocampal efferents, that interconnects the hippocampus of each cerebral hemisphere and the ipsilateral septal area and hypothalamus.
  Body. Upper arched cable formed by the union of the crura beneath the septa pellucida in the midline.
  Column. One of the two bundles that diverge from the body, then pass down and back toward the mammillary bodies.
  Crus. One of the two origins (legs) of the body, formed by detachment of the fimbria from the hippocampus.
  Fimbria. Hippocampal efferents that have assembled from the alveus on their way into the crus.
  Precommissural fornix. Fornix fibers that leave the columns just above the anterior commissure, bound for the septal nuclei, ventral striatum, and some nearby cortical areas.

Fourth ventricle. The most caudal of the brain ventricles, shaped like a tent with a peaked roof protruding into the overlying cerebellum and a diamond-shaped floor formed by the upper surface of the pons and rostral medulla; confluent with the third ventricle via the cerebral aqueduct and open to the subarachnoid space through three foramina: one median aperture and two lateral apertures.

Frontal lobe. The most anterior lobe of each cerebral hemisphere. The frontal lobe includes motor, premotor, and supplementary motor cortex; an extensive prefrontal region; and a large expanse of orbital cortex. The latter two regions have access via long association fibers to all other lobes and also the limbic system; they are important (in a poorly understood way) in regulating emotional tone, prioritizing bodily/environmental demands, and stabilizing short- and long-range goal-directed activity.

Globus pallidus. A wedge-shaped nucleus medial to the putamen that gives rise to most of the efferents from the basal ganglia.
  External segment. Afferents from the striatum and subthalamic nucleus, efferents (via the subthalamic fasciculus) to the subthalamic nucleus.
  Internal segment. Afferents from the striatum and subthalamic nucleus, efferents (via the ansa lenticularis and lenticular fasciculus) to the thalamus.

Glossopharyngeal nerve. The 9th cranial nerve. Its rootlets emerge laterally from a shallow groove on the lateral surface of the medulla. This nerve serves nasooropharyngeal, carotid body/sinus, middle ear, taste, and external ear sensations; assists with swallowing (stylopharyngeus muscle); and regulates salivation (parotid gland).

Gracile tubercle. A conspicuous swelling, just caudal to the obex, located dorsomedially on the lower medulla overlying the nucleus gracilis, which mediates that part of the posterior column–medial lemniscus pathway carrying tactile and proprioceptive information from the leg and lower body.

Great vein (great cerebral vein of Galen). A large unpaired vessel arising in the superior cistern by union of the two internal cerebral veins. During its short course it receives the basal veins (of Rosenthal), then turns superiorly around the splenium of the corpus callosum and joins the inferior sagittal sinus to form the straight sinus. The great vein is a key conduit in the deep venous drainage of the brain.

Gyrus rectus. A slender straight convolution that forms the most medial part of orbital cortex. Gyrus rectus has extensive limbic connections, particularly in circuits involving the amygdala.

Habenula. A small mound of neurons (derived from the embryonic diencephalon) on the dorsomedial surface of the caudal thalamus. The habenula receives diverse afferents from the mediobasal forebrain (e.g., septal nuclei, preoptic area) that arrive through the superiorly arching stria medullaris of the thalamus. Habenular efferents descend to various paramedian midbrain reticular nuclei via the habenulointerpeduncular tract. Hence it is anatomically evident that the habenula is a relay in caudally directed limbic projections, although its exact role is poorly understood.

Habenulointerpeduncular tract. (Also called *fasciculus retroflexus,* owing to its lordotic curvature), conveys output from the superiorly coursing stria medullaris/habenula route precipitously down again to the paramedian midbrain reticular formation (where all other caudally directed limbic projections arrive more expediently by passing inferiorly through the hypothalamus).

Heschl's gyri. See *transverse temporal gyri.*

Hippocampus. A specialized cortical area rolled into the medial temporal lobe. The hippocampus plays a critical role in the consolidation of new memories of facts and events. Anatomically, it has three subdivisions (until recently, usually referred to collectively as the *hippocampal formation* rather than the *hippocampus*), from within outward as follows:
  Dentate gyrus. In cross section, one of two interlocking C-shaped strips of cortex (the hippocampus proper is the other). Afferents from entorhinal cortex, efferents to hippocampal pyramidal cells.
  Hippocampus proper (also called *cornu ammonis,* or *Ammon's horn*). Afferents from the dentate gyrus and septal nuclei, efferents to the subiculum and septal nuclei.
  Subiculum. A transitional zone between the hippocampus proper and entorhinal cortex, the subiculum receives afferents from the hippocampus proper and is the principal source of efferents from the hippocampus in general.

Hypoglossal nerve. The 12th cranial nerve, whose rootlets emerge from the medulla in an anterolateral sulcus between the pyramid and the olive. It innervates intrinsic and extrinsic skeletal muscles of the tongue.

Hypoglossal nucleus. A group of lower motor neurons that innervate muscles of the ipsilateral half of the tongue.

Hypoglossal trigone. A triangular elevation in the floor of the caudal fourth ventricle formed by the underlying hypoglossal nucleus.

Hypothalamic sulcus. A shallow, curved indentation (convex side down) in the wall of the third ventricle, extending from the interventricular foramen to the opening of the cerebral aqueduct. The hypothalamic sulcus is the boundary between the thalamus and the hypothalamus.

Hypothalamus. The most inferior of the four longitudinal divisions of the diencephalon, the hypothalamus plays a major role in orchestrating visceral and drive-related activities. It has three general zones:

Anterior region. Includes the suprachiasmatic, supraoptic, and paraventricular nuclei; projects axons to the neurohypophysis and to caudal sites (including the spinal cord).

Tuberal region. Includes the dorsomedial, ventromedial, and arcuate nuclei. The latter secretes releasing hormones and inhibiting hormones into the pituitary portal system.

Posterior region. Includes the mammillary and posterior nuclei and projects to the thalamus and midbrain tegmentum.

Inferior brachium. See *brachium of the inferior colliculus.*

Inferior cerebellar peduncle. A major input route to the cerebellum, containing crossed olivocerebellar fibers, the uncrossed posterior spinocerebellar and cuneocerebellar tracts, vestibulocerebellar fibers, and other cerebellar afferents. Sometimes referred to as the restiform (Latin for "ropelike") body.

Inferior colliculus. A large, rounded mass of gray matter in the roof of the caudal midbrain. The inferior colliculus is a major link in the auditory system, receiving the lateral lemniscus and giving rise to the inferior brachium, which in turn conveys auditory fibers to the medial geniculate nucleus.

Inferior frontal gyrus. The most inferior of three longitudinally oriented frontal gyri. The opercular and triangular parts of this gyrus in the dominant hemisphere form Broca's area, which is a language area important for the production of spoken and written language.

Inferior olivary nucleus. A large nucleus in the anterolateral medulla, shaped like a bag, with a convoluted wall of gray matter (like a crumpled, pitted olive). Olivary afferents are diverse (from the spinal cord, red nucleus, deep cerebellar nuclei, etc.), but efferents are all olivocerebellar. They pour out of its medially facing mouth (or hilus), cross the midline as internal arcuate fibers, join the inferior cerebellar peduncle, and blanket the contralateral cerebellum as climbing fibers that powerfully excite Purkinje cells and other neurons.

Inferior parietal lobule. The lower part of the lateral surface of the parietal lobe, between the intraparietal and lateral sulci. The inferior parietal lobule consists of the angular and supramarginal gyri, which (in the dominant hemisphere) are functionally related to Wernicke's area and thus important in the comprehension of language.

Inferior temporal gyrus. The most inferior of three longitudinally oriented convolutions visible on the lateral aspect of the temporal lobe. The inferior temporal gyrus is part of a large region of visual association cortex occupying most of the occipital lobe and much of the temporal lobe.

Inferior thalamic peduncle. A small bundle of fibers emerging anteriorly from the thalamus and curving down toward the basal forebrain (just medial to the ansa lenticularis). Its fibers include interconnections between the dorsomedial nucleus and orbital cortex, but they do not traverse the internal capsule like other thalamic connections.

Infundibulum. The hollow, funnel-like stalk of the pituitary gland descending from the median eminence of the hypothalamus to the neurohypophysis. The infundibulum arises during embryonic development as a ventral outgrowth of the diencephalic floor, and is later joined by the adenohypophysis derived from the roof of the oral cavity.

Insula. The original lateral surface of the embryonic telencephalic vesicle overlying an area of fusion with the diencephalon, forming in the adult a central lobe of the cerebral hemisphere, typically convoluted into about three short gyri (located more anteriorly) and two long gyri. With rapid cerebral expansion during fetal development, the insula is overgrown and by birth concealed by frontal, parietal, and temporal opercula. It includes gustatory and autonomic areas, but is less well understood than other cortical areas because of its hidden location.

Internal arcuate fibers. A general term for the large collection of axons that arch across the midline of the medulla. Many internal arcuate fibers are axons leaving the posterior column nuclei to form the contralateral medial lemniscus; most others are olivocerebellar fibers.

Internal capsule. A compact, curved sheaf of thalamocortical, corticothalamic, and other cortical projection fibers shaped like part of a funnel. The internal capsule is divided into five regions, based on each region's relationship to the lenticular nucleus:

Anterior limb. Between the lenticular nucleus and the head of the caudate nucleus. Connections between the thalamus (dorsomedial and anterior nuclei) and prefrontal and anterior cingulate cortex, plus many frontopontine fibers.

Genu. At the junction between the anterior and posterior limbs. Connections between the thalamus (VA, VL) and motor/premotor cortex, plus some frontopontine fibers.

Posterior limb. Between the lenticular nucleus and the thalamus. Connections between the thalamus (VA, VL, VPL/VPM) and motor, somatosensory, and other parietal cortex, plus corticobulbar and corticospinal fibers.

Retrolenticular part. Passing posterior to the lenticular nucleus. Connections between the thalamus (pulvinar, LP) and parietal-occipital-temporal association cortex, plus the upper part of the optic radiation (from the lateral geniculate nucleus).

Sublenticular part. Dipping under the posterior part of the lenticular nucleus. Projections to and from the temporal lobe, including the auditory radiation (from the medial geniculate nucleus) and the lower part of the optic radiation (from the lateral geniculate nucleus) before it turns posteriorly toward the occipital lobe.

Internal carotid artery. A large distributing artery, originating from the bifurcation of the common carotid artery and running cranially in the neck to enter the base of the skull and eventually the cranial vault. The internal carotid artery branches at the circle of Willis into anterior and middle cerebral arteries. The paired carotids account for 85% of cerebral blood flow and thus supply most of the blood to the brain.

Internal cerebral vein. The major deep vein of each cerebral hemisphere, formed at the interventricular foramen by the confluence of the smaller septal and terminal (thalamostriate) veins (the latter receiving the choroidal vein, which drains much of the choroid plexus). Immediately after its origin the internal cerebral vein bends sharply posteriorly (through the venous angle), proceeds posteriorly in the transverse fissure, and fuses with its counterpart in the superior cistern to form the unpaired great vein.

Internal medullary lamina (of the thalamus). A dense, curved sheet of myelinated fibers within the thalamus that divide it into medial and lateral compartments everywhere except posteriorly, where it does not enter the pulvinar, and anteriorly, where it forks into a V-shaped groove for the anterior nuclei. The internal medullary lamina contains several small and two large intralaminar nuclei (the centromedian and parafascicular nuclei).

Interpeduncular fossa. A depression on the anterior aspect of the midbrain between the two cerebral peduncles. Its surface is penetrated by paramedian branches of the basilar artery and is therefore termed the *posterior perforated substance*. Rootlets of the oculomotor nerve exit here.

Interposed nucleus. The deep cerebellar nucleus interposed between the dentate and fastigial nuclei. The interposed nucleus has two distinct subdivisions, the globose nucleus medially and emboliform nucleus laterally (looks like an embolus in the hilus of the adjoining dentate nucleus). Both subdivisions receive input from the paravermal (intermediate) zone of cerebellar cortex, both project (via the superior cerebellar peduncle, like the dentate nucleus) to the red nucleus and ventral lateral nucleus of the thalamus. (The projection of the interposed nucleus differs mainly in emphasis, favoring the red nucleus over VL, whereas the dentate projection is just the opposite.)

Interthalamic adhesion (massa intermedia). A small, ovoid area of continuity between the two thalami resulting from expansion of the walls of the third ventricle during development and their fusion. The interthalamic adhesion is mainly gray matter, containing neurons and axonal and dendritic processes. (This structure is often reduced in size or absent, especially in the brains of elderly persons; however, in some mammals, such as rodents, it is massive, reducing the size of the third ventricle but anatomically making the thalamus almost a single unpaired structure.)

Interventricular foramen (of Monro). The narrow orifice between each lateral ventricle and the third ventricle.

Intraparietal sulcus. A longitudinally oriented sulcus on the lateral aspect of the parietal lobe, separating it into a superior parietal lobule above and an inferior parietal lobule below.

Lamina terminalis. A thin membrane at the anterior end of the third ventricle, curving down from the rostrum of the corpus callosum to the optic chiasm and corresponding (roughly, if not precisely) to the rostral end of the neural tube. The lamina terminalis connects the two telencephalic vesicles of the embryonic forebrain and provides a route through which commissural fibers that will later comprise the anterior commissure and corpus callosum begin to grow.

Lateral corticospinal tract. The larger of the two corticospinal tracts, comprising those fibers (about 85%) in each medullary pyramid that enter the pyramidal decussation and cross the midline to the opposite lateral funiculus. The axons of this tract end on spinal motor neurons or (more often) on smaller interneurons that in turn synapse on motor neurons. Its fibers are often said to be arranged somatotopically, with those passing to more caudal cord levels located more laterally, but anatomical evidence does not support this view.

Lateral cuneate nucleus. The equivalent for the arm of Clarke's nucleus for the leg. Proprioceptive primary afferents travel through fasciculus cuneatus to this nucleus, which then gives rise to uncrossed cuneocerebellar fibers that enter the cerebellum via the inferior cerebellar peduncle.

Lateral dorsal nucleus. See *thalamus*.

Lateral funiculus. One of the three major divisions of the spinal white matter, the others being the anterior and posterior funiculi. The lateral funiculus contains various ascending and descending tracts, including the spinocerebellar, spinothalamic, and lateral corticospinal tracts.

Lateral geniculate nucleus. See *thalamus*.

Lateral horn. A small, pointed lateral extension of the intermediate spinal gray noted from T1 through L2 or L3. The lateral horn contains the intermediolateral cell column, a long strand of preganglionic sympathetic neurons serving the entire body. Axons of these preganglionic sympathetic neurons leave through the ventral roots.

Lateral lemniscus. A flattened ribbon of fibers on the lateral surface of the rostral pontine tegmentum, arising from the cochlear nuclei and superior olivary complex. The lateral lemniscus is part of the ascending auditory pathway, conveying information from both ears to the inferior colliculus.

Lateral olfactory tract. A small tract (in humans) through which olfactory fibers travel across the surface of the basal forebrain to olfactory cortex and the amygdala.

Lateral posterior nucleus. See *thalamus*.

Lateral sulcus (Sylvian fissure). A long, deep fossa on the lateral aspect of each cerebral hemisphere resulting from downward and forward expansion of the temporal lobe during fetal development. The insula lies hidden within the depths of this sulcus, which separates the temporal lobe from the frontal and parietal lobes and provides a route by which the middle cerebral artery accesses the lateral convexity.

Lateral ventricle. The large central cavity of each cerebral hemisphere, following a C-shaped course throughout its extent and derived from the lumen of the embryonic telencephalic vesicle.

  Anterior horn. The frontal horn, in the frontal lobe anterior to the interventricular foramen.

  Body. In the frontal and parietal lobes, extending posteriorly to the region of the splenium of the corpus callosum.

  Atrium (or trigone). The region near the splenium where the body and the posterior and inferior horns meet.

  Inferior horn. The temporal horn, curving down and forward into the temporal lobe.

  Posterior horn. The occipital horn, projecting backward into the occipital lobe.

Lenticular fasciculus. Part of the projection from the globus pallidus to the thalamus. It has more axons than the other part (see *ansa lenticularis*) and is more spread out, forming numerous conspicuous bundles of myelinated fibers running medially through the internal capsule, like the teeth of a comb. Medial to the internal capsule the lenticular fasciculus is joined by the ansa lenticularis before both enter the thalamus.

Lenticular nucleus. The putamen and globus pallidus considered as one anatomical structure.

Lenticulostriate arteries. A collection of about a dozen small branches of the middle cerebral artery along its course toward the lateral sulcus. They penetrate the overlying brain near their origin and pass upward to supply deep structures (internal capsule, globus pallidus, putamen). The lenticulostriate arteries exemplify a large collection of small penetrating vessels that arise from all arteries around the base of the brain; these narrow, thin-walled vessels are involved frequently in strokes that deprive deep cerebral structures of blood and thus cause neurological deficits out of proportion to their size.

Limbic lobe. The most medial lobe of the cerebral hemisphere, facing the midline and visible grossly only in sagittal section. The limbic lobe consists of a continuous border zone of cortex around the corpus callosum, comprising the cingulate and parahippocampal gyri and their narrow connecting isthmus; this lobe and its many connections, cortical and subcortical, make up and characterize the limbic system.

Limen insulae. *Limen* is Latin for "threshold," and in this case refers to the transition point from anterior perforated substance to insula. The circular sulcus, which surrounds almost the entire insula, ends on either side of the limen insulae, allowing access for the middle cerebral artery.

Lingual gyrus. The gyrus forming the inferior bank of the calcarine sulcus. The lingual gyrus overlaps the posterior portion of the occipitotemporal gyrus, separated from it by the collateral sulcus.

Lissauer's tract. A pale-staining area of white matter between the substantia gelatinosa (capping the posterior gray horn of the spinal cord) and the pial surface of the cord. Lissauer's tract stains more lightly than the rest of the spinal white matter because it contains finely myelinated and unmyelinated pain and temperature fibers (derived from the lateral division of each dorsal root filament) which then distribute into the underlying gelatinosa over several segments.

Locus ceruleus. A column of pigmented, blue-black neurons (*locus ceruleus* is Latin for "blue spot") near the floor of the fourth ventricle, extending through the rostral pons. Locus ceruleus neurons provide most of the far-flung noradrenergic innervation of the cerebrum.

Longitudinal fissure. An extensive vertical cleft, oriented sagittally and occupied by the falx cerebri, separating the two cerebral hemispheres around the margin of the undivided corpus callosum.

Mammillary body. A prominent component of the posterior hypothalamus. The mammillary body receives afferents from the hippocampus (chiefly the subiculum) via the fornix, and sends efferents to the anterior nucleus of the thalamus via the mammillothalamic tract. This is part of a historic neural circuit proposed by James Papez in 1937 as an anatomical substrate for emotion. Although derided by some then and viewed as simplistic by others now, the Papez circuit—a grand loop from hippocampus through hypothalamus, thalamus, and cortex back to hippocampus again—was unquestionably the impetus for the decades of research that led to the limbic system concept of today.

Mammillothalamic tract. The projection from the mammillary body to the anterior nucleus of the thalamus; part of the Papez circuit.

Medial geniculate nucleus. See *thalamus.*

Medial lemniscus. Somatosensory afferents originating from the contralateral posterior column nuclei and trigeminal main sensory nucleus and ascending through the brainstem to the thalamus (VPL/VPM). The medial lemniscus is the principal ascending pathway for tactile and proprioceptive information.

Medial longitudinal fasciculus (MLF). A longitudinal fiber bundle involved in coordinating eye and head movements. The MLF includes fibers from contralateral abducens interneurons to medial rectus motor neurons in the oculomotor nucleus. It is also the route of descent for fibers of the medial vestibulospinal tract.

Medial striate artery. A large penetrating branch of the anterior cerebral artery, also known as the *recurrent artery of Heubner.* It supplies the striatum in the region of nucleus accumbens and also the anterior limb and genu of the internal capsule.

Median aperture. One of the three apertures through which the fourth ventricle communicates with subarachnoid space. The median aperture (also called the *foramen of Magendie*) opens into cisterna magna.

Medulla (medulla oblongata). The most caudal of the three subdivisions of the brainstem, continuous rostrally with the pons and caudally with the spinal cord. This small structure is important out of proportion to its size: it is crucial to vital functions (respiratory, cardiovascular, visceral activity) and other integrative activities; most sensory and motor tracts of the CNS run up and down through it.

Midbrain (mesencephalon). The most rostral of the three subdivisions of the brainstem. The midbrain remains tubular in plan but features a great variety of structures: the superior and inferior colliculi in its roof (tectum), aqueduct and periaqueductal gray, oculomotor and trochlear nuclei and pretectal area, upper part of the reticular formation, red nuclei, substantia nigra, and cerebral peduncles. Like the medulla, a small region of enormous importance.

Middle cerebellar peduncle. The largest of the cerebellar peduncles, containing fibers from contralateral pontine nuclei that end as mossy fibers in almost all areas of cerebellar cortex. Sometimes referred to as the *brachium pontis* (the "arm of the pons").

Middle cerebral artery. The more posterior of the two terminal branches of the internal carotid. The middle cerebral artery runs laterally beneath the basal forebrain to reach the lateral sulcus, where many branches arise. It supplies the insula, most of the lateral surface of the cerebral hemisphere, and the anterior tip of the temporal lobe.

Middle frontal gyrus. One of three longitudinally oriented frontal gyri, situated between the superior and inferior frontal gyri. It includes part of premotor cortex, as well as the frontal eye field, which is involved in initiating voluntary eye movements to the contralateral side.

Middle temporal gyrus. One of three longitudinally oriented gyri on the lateral surface of the temporal lobe between the superior and inferior temporal gyri. It contains some visual association cortex, as well as multimodal or heteromodal association cortex.

MLF. See *medial longitudinal fasciculus.*

Nucleus accumbens. The most inferior part of the striatum, with predominantly limbic connections. Nucleus accumbens was traditionally known as *nucleus accumbens septi* but is now recognized as a major component of the ventral striatum. (The original, longer name reflects its position immediately lateral to the base of the septum pellucidum, as if leaning against it.)

Nucleus ambiguus. A collection of lower motor neurons for laryngeal and pharyngeal muscles, and preganglionic parasympathetic neurons for the heart.

Nucleus cuneatus. Site of termination of fasciculus cuneatus and origin of the arm region of the medial lemniscus.

Nucleus gracilis. Site of termination of fasciculus gracilis and origin of the leg region of the medial lemniscus.

Nucleus of the solitary tract. The principal visceral sensory nucleus of the brainstem; the site of termination of the visceral primary afferents in the solitary tract.

Obex. Apex of the V-shaped caudal fourth ventricle, where the ventricle narrows into the central canal of the lower medulla and spinal cord.

Occipital lobe. The most posterior lobe of each cerebral hemisphere. The occipital lobe includes the primary visual cortex on the banks of the calcarine sulcus, as well as adjoining areas of visual association cortex.

Occipitotemporal gyrus (fusiform gyrus). A long gyrus, beginning just lateral to the uncus and running posteriorly along the inferior surface of the temporal lobe to the occipital lobe. Along its course in the temporal lobe the occipitotemporal gyrus is bounded laterally by the inferior temporal gyrus and medially by the parahippocampal gyrus.

Oculomotor nerve. The 3rd cranial nerve, emerging into the interpeduncular fossa of the midbrain. The oculomotor nerve innervates most of the extrinsic ocular muscles (see also *oculomotor nucleus*): superior, medial, and inferior recti, inferior oblique, and levator palpebrae superioris. It also conveys preganglionic parasympathetic fibers to the ciliary ganglion, where postganglionic fibers arise to innervate the pupillary sphincter and ciliary muscle.

Oculomotor nucleus. Lower motor neurons for the ipsilateral medial and inferior recti and inferior oblique, the contralateral superior rectus, and the levator palpebrae of both sides. Preganglionic parasympathetic neurons in one of its columns, the Edinger-Westphal nucleus, control the ipsilateral pupillary sphincter and ciliary muscle.

Olfactory bulb. The knoblike anterior end of the olfactory tract on the orbital surface of the frontal lobe. The olfactory bulb is the site of central termination of incoming olfactory fibers from the olfactory epithelium in the nasal cavity. It is large and well laminated in animals depending heavily upon the sense of smell, but relatively small and poorly differentiated in the human brain.

Olfactory sulcus. A sulcus on the orbital surface of the frontal lobe, immediately lateral to gyrus rectus and harboring the olfactory bulb and tract.

Olfactory tract. Projections from olfactory bulb neurons (mitral and tufted cells) to olfactory (piriform) cortex and the amygdala. The olfactory tract also conveys modulatory efferents traveling from deeper olfactory centers back to the olfactory bulb.

Olfactory tubercle. A restricted area of the anterior perforated substance where some olfactory tract fibers terminate. The olfactory tubercle forms a distinct elevation in some animals, but is not very apparent in human brains.

Olive. Protuberance on the lateral aspect of the medulla, just dorsolateral to the pyramid, caused by the underlying inferior olivary nucleus.

Opercula (singular, operculum). The parts of the frontal, parietal, and temporal lobes bordering the lateral sulcus and overlying the insula, hiding it from view.

Opercular part (inferior frontal gyrus). The most caudal part of the inferior frontal gyrus, containing the caudal half of Broca's area (see *inferior frontal gyrus*).

Optic chiasm. The site at which optic nerve fibers from ganglion cells in the nasal half of each retina decussate, so that each optic tract contains fibers arising in the temporal retina of the ipsilateral eye and the nasal retina of the opposite eye.

Optic nerve. The 2nd cranial nerve, containing axons of the various types of retinal ganglion cells projecting to the lateral geniculate nucleus of the thalamus, superior colliculus, pretectal area, suprachiasmatic nucleus of the hypothalamus, and a few other sites.

Optic radiation. A conspicuous, sharply defined, and heavily myelinated bundle of visual fibers originating in the lateral geniculate nucleus, departing the thalamus through the retrolenticular and sublenticular parts of the internal capsule, curving in a broad fan around the atrium and the posterior and inferior horns of the lateral ventricle, and terminating in the primary visual cortex on the upper and lower banks of the calcarine sulcus.

Optic tract. Axons of ganglion cells from corresponding (homonymous) halves of each retina on their way to the lateral geniculate nucleus, superior colliculus, pretectal area, and a few other sites.

Orbital gyri. The variably sulcated (in a pattern often resembling the letter H) group of gyri that comprise the orbital surface of the frontal lobe. The orbital gyri are not named individually, in contrast to the gyrus rectus immediately medial to them. (The gyrus rectus is on the orbital surface, but is usually not included among the orbital gyri.)

Orbital part (inferior frontal gyrus). The most anterior of the various frontal folds covering the insula, so named because it merges with the orbital gyri.

Parafascicular nucleus. See *thalamus*.

Parabrachial nucleus. A collection of nuclei adjacent to the superior cerebellar peduncle (brachium conjunctivum) as the latter traverses the rostral pons. Various parts of the parabrachial nucleus are involved in transferring visceral sensory information to the hypothalamus and amygdala.

Paracentral lobule. The extensions of the precentral and postcentral gyri onto the medial surface of the hemisphere, forming a lobule that surrounds the end of the central sulcus.

Parahippocampal gyrus. The gyrus immediately adjacent to the hippocampus. Its anterior region contains the entorhinal cortex, a meeting ground for cortical projections from multiple areas and the source of most afferents to the hippocampus.

Parietal lobe. A cerebral lobe bounded by the frontal, temporal, and occipital lobes on the lateral surface of each hemisphere, and by the frontal, limbic, and occipital lobes on the medial surface. The parietal lobe contains primary somatosensory cortex in the postcentral gyrus, areas involved in language comprehension (in the inferior parietal lobule, usually on the left), and regions involved in complex aspects of spatial orientation and perception.

Parietooccipital sulcus. A deep fissure separating the parietal and occipital lobes on the medial aspect of the cerebral hemisphere. Inferiorly the parietooccipital sulcus joins the calcarine sulcus, which continues into the temporal lobe as a common stem for both these sulci.

Periamygdaloid cortex. A cortical area covering part of the amygdala and merging with it; part of primary olfactory cortex.

Periaqueductal gray. An area of gray matter and poorly myelinated fibers surrounding the aqueduct in the midbrain. The periaqueductal gray is the site of origin of a descending pain-control pathway that relays in nucleus raphe magnus (among other connections).

Pineal gland. A dorsal outgrowth of the diencephalon, protruding from the third ventricle immediately caudal to the paired habenular nuclei. The pineal is an endocrine gland important in seasonal cycles of some animals, but its function in humans is not yet clear.

Piriform cortex. A cortical area overlying the lateral olfactory tract as moves toward the temporal lobe; part of primary olfactory cortex.

Pons. The second of the three parts of the brainstem, continuous rostrally with the midbrain and caudally with the medulla. The pons is overlain by the cerebellum and includes an enlarged basal region (see *basal pons*).

Pontine nuclei. A collective term for the many small nuclei in the basal pons that receive afferents from cerebral cortex (via the internal capsule and cerebral peduncle) and project to contralateral cerebellar cortex (via the middle cerebellar peduncle).

Pontocerebellar fibers. Projections from pontine nuclei to the contralateral cerebellar cortex, where they terminate as mossy fibers (as do all cerebellar afferents except those from the inferior olivary nucleus).

Postcentral gyrus. A vertically oriented convolution of the parietal lobe immediately posterior to the central sulcus. The postcentral gyrus is the site of primary somatosensory cortex.

Posterior cerebral artery. A prominent artery that arises from the bifurcation of the basilar artery at the level of the midbrain. The posterior cerebral artery forms the caudal part of the circle of Willis and supplies the rostral midbrain, posterior thalamus, medial occipital lobe, and inferior and medial surfaces of the temporal lobe.

Posterior column. The entire contents of one posterior funiculus except for its share of the propriospinal tract (a thin shell of white matter around the gray matter).

Posterior commissure. Crossing fibers interconnecting the two sides of the rostral midbrain and pretectal area. These crossing fibers are involved in the consensual pupillary light reflex and in coordinating vertical eye movements.

Posterior communicating artery. A short vessel connecting the posterior cerebral artery to the internal carotid, thereby forming one link in the circle of Willis. Normally pressures in the internal carotid and posterior cerebral arteries are balanced so that little or no blood flows around the circle, but if one vessel is occluded the posterior communicating artery may allow anastomotic flow and thus prevent neurologic damage.

Posterior funiculus. One of the three major divisions of the spinal white matter, principally occupied by ascending collaterals of large myelinated primary afferents carrying impulses from various kinds of mechanoreceptors. This is the first stage of the major pathway to cerebral cortex for low-threshold cutaneous, joint, and muscle receptor information.

Posterior inferior cerebellar artery. A long, circumferential branch of the vertebral artery, supplying much of the inferior surface of the cerebellar hemisphere; en route it sends shorter branches to the choroid plexus of the fourth ventricle and to much of the lateral medulla; referred to by the acronym PICA.

Posterior spinocerebellar tract. Uncrossed fibers from Clarke's nucleus, carrying proprioceptive information from the arm to the ipsilateral half of the cerebellar vermis and intermediate zone via the inferior cerebellar peduncle.

Precentral gyrus. A vertically oriented convolution of the frontal lobe immediately anterior to the central sulcus. The precentral gyrus is the site of primary motor cortex.

Precuneus. The part of the parietal lobe on the medial surface of the hemisphere, excluding the medial extension of the postcentral gyrus.

Preoccipital notch. The midpoint of a shallow, curved indentation along the inferior margin of the lateral aspect of each cerebral hemisphere. The preoccipital notch serves as a landmark for synthesizing boundaries for the parietal, occipital, and temporal lobes on the lateral and medial surfaces of hemisphere.

Preoptic region. The area in the walls of the third ventricle immediately anterior to the optic chiasm; technically a telencephalic region but structurally and functionally continuous with the hypothalamus of the diencephalon.

Pretectal area. The region between the superior colliculus and caudal thalamus. The pretectal area receives afferents from the retina and visual association cortex. It projects efferents bilaterally to the Edinger-Westphal nuclei, crossing both in the posterior commissure and in the ventral periaqueductal gray. It is important in the pupillary light reflex.

Pulvinar. See *thalamus*.

Putamen. The part of the striatum involved most prominently in the motor functions of the basal ganglia. The putamen receives afferents from cerebral cortex (primarily motor and somatosensory areas), and from the substantia nigra (compact part) and thalamic centromedian nucleus. It projects efferents to the globus pallidus, which in turn projects via the thalamus (VA, VL) to premotor and supplementary motor areas. The putamen forms the outer component of the lenticular nucleus (the globus pallidus is the inner part).

Pyramid. Corticospinal fibers from the ipsilateral precentral gyrus and adjacent areas of cerebral cortex, forming a prominent fiber bundle (roughly triangular in cross section, which gave rise to the name) on the ventral surface of the medulla.

Pyramidal decussation. The site, located at the spinomedullary junction, at which most fibers in each pyramid cross the midline to form the contralateral lateral corticospinal tract.

Raphe nuclei. A series of nuclei extending through the brainstem near the midline of the tegmentum, collectively providing the serotoninergic innervation of the CNS.

Red nucleus. The site of termination of part of the superior cerebellar peduncle, and the site of origin of uncrossed fibers to the inferior olivary nucleus and of the crossed rubrospinal tract.

Reticular formation. The central region of the brainstem, forming the tegmentum of the midbrain, pons, and medulla, with a complex netlike fabric of nerve cell bodies and interwoven processes; its myriad multimodal afferents, profusely collateralizing efferents running upward and downward to every level of the CNS, and involvement in virtually every activity from visceral functions to consciousness make it a core integrating structure of the brain.

Reticular nucleus. See *thalamus*.

Rhinal sulcus. A sulcus demarcating the anterior boundary of the uncus on the medial aspect of the temporal lobe; sometimes continuous with the collateral sulcus behind it.

Septal nuclei. A component of the medial wall of the cerebral hemisphere just beneath the base of the largely glial septum pellucidum. The septal nuclei are continuous inferiorly with the preoptic area and hypothalamus and are reciprocally connected with the hippocampus, amygdala, hypothalamus, and other limbic structures via the fornix, stria terminalis, and other tracts. They are also the source of cholinergic input to the hippocampus.

Septal vein. A deep cerebral vein that runs posteriorly across the septum pellucidum to join the thalamostriate (terminal) vein and thus form the internal cerebral vein.

Septum pellucidum. A thin, chiefly glial, almost transparent, paired membrane separating the two lateral ventricles. (In most brains the two septa pellucida are so closely apposed as to appear as a single structure, and for simplicity they are so labeled in most of the illustrations in this book.)

Solitary tract. Primary afferents conveying visceral information from cranial nerves VII, IX, and X to the adjacent solitary nucleus surrounding the tract.

Spinothalamic tract. Crossed fibers from neurons in the posterior horn of the spinal cord conveying pain and temperature information to the thalamus (VPL).

Stria medullaris (of the thalamus). The site of attachment of the roof of the third ventricle and a route through which septal efferents reach the habenula.

Stria terminalis. A slender, poorly myelinated tract following a long C-shaped course within the thalamostriate groove that separates the caudate nucleus from the thalamus. The stria terminalis plays a role analogous to that played by the fornix for the hippocampus—it conveys efferents from the amygdala to the septal area and hypothalamus.

Striatum. An inclusive term for the caudate nucleus, putamen, and ventral striatum.

Stripe of Gennari. A sheet of myelinated fibers that run through one of the middle layers of primary visual cortex, giving it the distinctive appearance that gave rise to its alternate name, *striate cortex*. Named for the medical student who first described it in the 18th century.

Strumus (commonly misspelled *strumous*). A primitive telencephalic extension that, unlike structures such as the neocortex that have expanded greatly in primates, has remained constant in size and position. It is located rostral to the lamina terminalis, medial to gyrus rectus, and ventromedial to the substantia innominata. Only the anterior and ventral nuclear groups are developed in humans, and these are subdivided cytoarchitectonically into four discrete nuclei: the anteroventral, anterior ventral, and the subdivided anterior and ventral ventral anterior nuclei.

The interconnections of the strumus are extensive and complex, but their importance cannot be underestimated. There are four major afferent pathways: a substantial input from a variably present limbic nucleus, the effluvium, traveling through the superior and inferior effluviostrumular tracts; and minor inputs from the trivium and nimbus in the temporal lobe. Because the strumus has no known efferent pathways, however, its functional importance has been difficult to justify anatomically. (The frequently mentioned strumulotrivionimboeffluviostrumular loop apparently does not exist.)

The clinical importance of the strumus is based on the disorder *subacute combined strumuloma*. This is an idiopathic disease of exquisitely rare occurrence and indeterminate symptomatology, which forms the basis for the identification of the strumus as the center controlling involuntary higher cortical functions.

Subcallosal fasciculus. A compact group of lightly-staining myelinated fibers in the white matter of each cerebral hemisphere (visible mainly in the frontal lobe). The subcallosal fasciculus forms a pale, arched band subjacent to the corpus callosum. It conveys inputs from cortex (chiefly association areas) to the caudate nucleus.

Substantia gelatinosa. A distinctive region of gray matter, surmounted by Lissauer's tract, that caps the posterior horn of the spinal cord at all levels. The substantia gelatinosa looks pale in myelin-stained material because its inputs are poorly myelinated or unmyelinated. It deals mostly with pain and temperature sensation.

Substantia nigra. A large nucleus in the midbrain, interposed between the red nucleus and cerebral peduncle. The substantia nigra has two parts: a compact part, containing closely packed, pigmented (with neuromelanin) dopaminergic neurons that project to the striatum, and a reticular part, containing more loosely arranged neurons, receiving inputs from the striatum and projecting to the thalamus.

Subthalamic fasciculus. Small bundles of fibers that cross the internal capsule like the teeth of a comb. Fibers of the subthalamic fasciculus interconnect the globus pallidus and subthalamic nucleus, which face each other on either side of the internal capsule.

Subthalamic nucleus. A lens-shaped, biconvex mass of gray matter just medial and superior to the junction of the internal capsule and cerebral peduncle. The subthalamic nucleus is the substrate of an indirect route through the basal ganglia: striatum → globus pallidus (external segment) → subthalamic nucleus → globus pallidus (internal segment) → thalamus. The globus pallidus–subthalamic nucleus connections travel in the subthalamic fasciculus.

Sulcus limitans. A longitudinal groove in the embryonic neural tube that separates sensory nuclei from motor nuclei. In the adult brain it persists as a groove in the floor of the fourth ventricle that separates motor nuclei of cranial nerves (medial to it) from sensory nuclei of cranial nerves.

Superior brachium. See *brachium of the superior colliculus.*

Superior cerebellar artery. A branch of the basilar artery that arises just caudal to its bifurcation. Long circumferential branches supply the superior surface of the cerebellum, and shorter branches supply much of the rostral pons and caudal midbrain.

Superior cerebellar peduncle. The major efferent route from the cerebellum, containing projections from deep cerebellar nuclei on their way to the red nucleus and VL. Sometimes referred to as the *brachium conjunctivum* (a "joined-together arm," named for its course through a decussation with its contralateral counterpart).

Superior cistern. The enlarged, CSF-filled subarachnoid cistern above the midbrain, also termed the *quadrigeminal cistern* and the *cistern of the great cerebral vein*. The superior cistern is an important radiological landmark, continuous anteriorly and posteriorly with the transverse fissure and laterally with thin, curved spaces that partially encircle the midbrain before joining its underlying interpeduncular cistern. (The combination of superior cistern and these sheetlike extensions is known as the *ambient cistern*.)

Superior colliculus. A large, rounded mass of gray matter in the roof of the rostral midbrain. The superior colliculus receives afferents from the retina and visual cortex, sends efferents to the pulvinar and other structures, and plays a role in visual attention and control of eye movements.

Superior frontal gyrus. The most superior of three longitudinally oriented frontal gyri, continuing onto the medial surface of the hemisphere. The superior frontal gyrus includes supplementary motor cortex and part of premotor cortex.

Superior olivary nucleus. A complex of nuclei near the rostral end of the facial motor nucleus in the caudal pons. The superior olivary nucleus is the first site of convergence of fibers representing the two ears and is the source of many fibers of the lateral lemniscus. It is also the origin of the crossed olivocochlear bundle that runs centrifugally in the contralateral cochlear nerve and terminates in the organ of Corti, modulating hair cell activity.

Superior parietal lobule. The upper part of the lateral surface of the parietal lobe, above the intraparietal sulcus. The superior parietal lobule contains somatosensory association cortex.

Superior temporal gyrus. The uppermost gyrus of the temporal lobe, bordering on the lateral sulcus. The superior temporal gyrus includes primary auditory cortex (actually located in the wall of the lateral sulcus, in transverse temporal gyri crossing the top of the superior temporal gyrus), auditory association cortex, and (usually on the left) Wernicke's area. This is one example of a region of visibly different size and configuration in the two cerebral hemispheres, typically being more extensive in the left hemisphere.

Supramarginal gyrus. The part of the inferior parietal lobule surrounding the up-turned end of the lateral sulcus. Although variable in size and shape, the supramarginal gyrus is important in language function.

Tegmentum. A general anatomical term for the area anterior to the ventricular spaces of the medulla, pons, and midbrain. Tegmentum is a useful umbrella term (Latin for "covering") for all structures covering the basal components of the brainstem (pyramids, basal pons, bases of cerebral peduncles) and includes the reticular formation, nuclei of cranial nerves, most ascending and descending tracts, the red nuclei and substantia nigra.

Temporal lobe. The most inferior lobe of each cerebral hemisphere, inferior to the lateral sulcus and anterior to the occipital lobe. The temporal lobe includes auditory sensory and association cortex, part of posterior language cortex, visual and higher-order association cortex, primary and association olfactory cortex, the amygdala and the hippocampus. (The parahippocampal gyrus, a major part of the limbic lobe, is also commonly referred to as part of the medial temporal lobe.)

Terminal vein. A deep cerebral vein traveling with the stria terminalis in the groove between the thalamus and adjacent caudate nucleus. It drains much of these two structures. See also *thalamostriate vein*.

Thalamostriate vein. A frequently used alternate name for the terminal vein, more useful because it says not only where the vessel is, but also what it does.

Thalamic fasciculus. Projections from the cerebellum (via the superior cerebellar peduncle) and basal ganglia (via the ansa and fasciculus lenticularis), gathered together beneath the ventral anterior and ventral lateral nuclei (VA/VL).

Thalamus. A collection of nuclei that collectively are the source of most extrinsic afferents to the cerebral cortex. Some thalamic nuclei (relay nuclei) receive distinct input bundles and project to discrete functional areas of the cerebral cortex. Others (association nuclei) are primarily interconnected with association cortex. Still others have diffuse cortical projections, and one has no projections to the cortex at all.

Anterior nucleus. The thalamic relay for the limbic system. Afferents from the mammillary body and other limbic structures, efferents to the cingulate gyrus.

Centromedian nucleus (CM). The largest intralaminar nucleus; afferents from the globus pallidus, efferents to the striatum (with branches projecting diffusely to widespread cortical areas).

Dorsomedial nucleus (DM). Interconnections with prefrontal association cortex and the limbic system.

Lateral dorsal nucleus. Efferents to the posterior part of the cingulate gyrus; in many ways an extension of the anterior nucleus.

Lateral geniculate nucleus (LGN). The thalamic relay for vision. Afferents from the retina via the optic tract, efferents to primary visual cortex above and below the calcarine sulcus.

Lateral posterior nucleus (LP). Interconnections, similar to those of the pulvinar, with posterior association cortex.

Medial geniculate nucleus (MGN). The thalamic relay for hearing. Afferents from the inferior colliculus via the inferior brachium, efferents to auditory cortex in the superior temporal gyrus.

Parafascicular nucleus (PF). An intralaminar nucleus with connections similar to those of the centromedian nucleus.

Pulvinar. The largest thalamic nucleus, interconnected with parietal-occipital-temporal association cortex.

Reticular nucleus. An unusual thalamic nucleus with no projections to the cortex. Afferents from the thalamus and cerebral cortex, GABAergic efferents back to the thalamus.

Ventral anterior nucleus (VA). A thalamic relay for the motor system. Afferents from the cerebellum and basal ganglia, efferents to motor areas of cortex.

Ventral lateral nucleus (VL). A thalamic relay for the motor system. Afferents from the cerebellum and basal ganglia, efferents to motor areas of cortex.

Ventral posterolateral nucleus (VPL). The thalamic relay for somatic sensation from the body. Afferents from the medial lemniscus and spinothalamic tract, efferents to somatosensory cortex in the postcentral gyrus.

Ventral posteromedial nucleus (VPM). The thalamic relay for somatic sensation from the head and for taste. Afferents from the trigeminal portions of the medial lemniscus and spinothalamic tract and from the nucleus of the solitary tract; efferents to somatosensory cortex in the postcentral gyrus and to gustatory cortex in and near the insula.

Third ventricle. The single, median, vertically oriented cavity of the diencephalon, separating the thalamus and hypothalamus of the two hemispheres. The third ventricle is confluent anteriorly with both lateral ventricles through the interventricular foramina and posteriorly with the aqueduct, and has four small outpocketings:

Infundibular recess. Leads into the hollow infundibular stalk.

Optic recess. Small recess just above and anterior to the optic chiasm.

Pineal recess. Leads into the stalk of the pineal gland.

Suprapineal recess. An outpocketing of the roof of the third ventricle just anterior to the pineal gland.

Transverse fissure. An extension of subarachnoid space, situated above the roof of the third ventricle and containing the internal cerebral veins. We use the term in a more extended sense in this book, to refer to the long slit intervening between the cerebral hemispheres and structures below them—the cleft normally occupied by the tentorium cerebelli, continuing into the superior cistern and from there into the subarachnoid space above the roof of the third ventricle.

Transverse temporal (Heschl's) gyri. Gyri (usually two in number) that run transversely across the lower bank of the lateral sulcus. The location of primary auditory cortex.

Trapezoid body. Auditory fibers from the cochlear nuclei to the superior olivary nucleus that cross the midline in a trapezoid-shaped area of the pontine tegmentum.

Triangular part (inferior frontal gyrus). The middle of the three parts of the inferior frontal gyrus, containing the anterior half of Broca's area (see *inferior frontal gyrus*).

Trigeminal nerve. The 5th cranial nerve, emerging anterolaterally from the basal pons. The trigeminal nerve conveys somatosensory (and some chemosensory) fibers from the ipsilateral half of the head, as well as efferents to ipsilateral muscles of mastication.

Motor root. Small, anterior root containing efferent fibers that distribute through the mandibular division of the nerve.

Sensory root. Massive, posterior root containing afferent fibers that arrive over all three divisions of the nerve.

Trigeminal nuclei.

Main sensory. Termination site of large-diameter afferents (the equivalent of a posterior column nucleus for the trigeminal system). Most of its efferents project to the contralateral VPM via the medial lemniscus; some, however, project to the ipsilateral VPM via the dorsal trigeminal tract.

Mesencephalic. The cell bodies of primary afferents from muscle spindles in muscles of mastication and from other oral mechanoreceptors.

Motor. Lower motor neurons for ipsilateral muscles of mastication.

Spinal. The termination site of the spinal trigeminal tract. The most caudal part of the nucleus (in the caudal medulla) looks like the spinal posterior horn, has a component similar to the substantia gelatinosa, and processes pain and temperature information. Its efferents project to VPM through the spinothalamic tract.

Trigeminal tracts.

Mesencephalic. Processes of cell bodies in the adjacent mesencephalic trigeminal nucleus that send one branch to innervate mechanoreceptors in and around the mouth, and others to central termination sites such as the main sensory nucleus.

Spinal. Central processes of primary afferents from the ipsilateral side of the face, conveying information about pain and temperature (and some tactile information).

Trochlear nerve. The 4th cranial nerve, emerging as an already-crossed small bundle from the posterior aspect of the midbrain, just caudal to the inferior colliculus. The trochlear nerve innervates the superior oblique muscle, which helps to intort the eyeball and turn it downward and laterally.

Trochlear nucleus. Lower motor neurons for the contralateral superior oblique muscle, located in the caudal midbrain just caudal to the oculomotor nucleus. Trochlear axons exit the paired nuclei, turn caudally in the overlying periaqueductal gray, arch posteriorly to decussate (like old-time ice tongs used to handle large blocks of ice), and leave the brainstem at the pons–midbrain junction.

Tuber cinereum. A low mound of gray matter on the inferior aspect of the hypothalamus, bounded by the optic chiasm, optic tracts, and anterior edge of the mammillary bodies. The tuber cinereum contains the median eminence and the beginning of the infundibular stalk and is a region of great importance in hypothalamic hormonal regulation of the adenohypophysis.

Uncus. A medial protuberance from the anterior end of the parahippocampal gyrus caused by the underlying amygdala. The proximity of its surface to the adjacent cerebral peduncle can cause clinical problems during cerebral edema or as a result of space-occupying masses.

Vagal trigone. A small elevation in the floor of the caudal fourth ventricle with boundaries forming a narrow triangle just lateral to the hypoglossal trigone. Each vagal trigone is a fusiform swelling produced by the underlying dorsal motor nucleus of the vagus.

Vagus nerve. The 10th cranial nerve, emerging as a series of filaments from a groove dorsal to the olive. The vagus has diverse components: efferents to branchial arch muscles arise from nucleus ambiguus in the medulla and mediate swallowing and phonation; efferents to parasympathetic ganglia for thoracic and abdominal viscera arise from the dorsal motor nucleus of the vagus and nucleus ambiguus in the medulla; afferent fibers mediate general visceral sensation, taste from the epiglottis, and cutaneous sensation behind the ear.

Vein of Galen. See *great vein*.

Venous angle. The point at which the newly formed internal cerebral vein turns sharply caudally as it leaves the interventricular foramen. This is an important radiological landmark indicating the location of the genu of the internal capsule and the anterior end of the thalamus.

Ventral amygdalofugal pathway. A massive but loosely organized fiber bundle running transversely in the basal forebrain. It interconnects the amygdala with the hypothalamus, septal area, thalamus, and even the brainstem, and is thus an important pathway of the limbic system.

Ventral anterior nucleus. See *thalamus*.

Ventral lateral nucleus. See *thalamus*.

Ventral pallidum. A limbic extension of the globus pallidus, located beneath the anterior commissure, with inputs from the ventral striatum. The ventral pallidum is part of a basal ganglia circuit similar to that involved in motor functions, but in this case has limbic inputs (amygdala, hippocampus ➡ ventral striatum ➡ ventral pallidum) and outputs (via the dorsomedial nucleus of the thalamus) to prefrontal and orbital cortex.

Ventral posterolateral nucleus. See *thalamus*.

Ventral posteromedial nucleus. See *thalamus*.

Ventral root. The anterior motor root of a spinal nerve, coalescing from a variable number of unevenly spaced rootlets that depart the spinal cord along its anterolateral sulcus.

Ventral striatum. The primarily limbic subdivision of the striatum, comprising nucleus accumbens, adjacent parts of the caudate nucleus and putamen, and certain nearby parts of the basal forebrain.

Ventral tegmental area. An unpaired region of the midbrain medial to the compact part of the substantia nigra, containing dopaminergic neurons that project to various limbic and neocortical areas.

Vermis. Midline, sinuous (*vermis* is Latin for "worm") zone of the cerebellum between the two cerebellar hemispheres. The vermis includes a representation of the trunk conveyed by the spinocerebellar tracts; its outputs, primarily through the fastigial nucleus, reach the vestibular nuclei and reticular formation.

Vertebral artery. One of the two major arteries that supply each side of the CNS (see also *internal carotid artery*). The vertebral artery originates as the first branch of the subclavian, runs cranially through foramina in cervical vertebrae, enters the base of the skull through the foramen magnum, and ascends along the medulla. At the pontomedullary junction it unites with its contralateral counterpart to form the basilar artery. The vertebral artery and its posterior inferior cerebellar branch (PICA) supply blood to the medulla and inferior part of the cerebellum, and it supplies the cervical spinal cord via the posterior and anterior spinal arteries.

Vestibular nuclei. Four elaborately subdivided secondary sensory nuclei of the vestibular division of the 8th cranial nerve in the floor of the fourth ventricle; collectively they project to the nuclei of extraocular muscles (mostly via the medial longitudinal fasciculus), the cerebellum, the reticular formation, and the spinal cord:

Inferior. Peppered with small bundles of vestibular primary afferents that run through it.

Lateral. Origin of the lateral vestibulospinal tract to ipsilateral extensor motor neurons.

Medial. Origin of the medial vestibulospinal tract, projecting bilaterally to cervical motor neurons.

Superior. Ascending and descending connections with nuclei of extraocular muscles (other vestibular nuclei also share in this).

Vestibulocochlear nerve. The 8th cranial nerve, emerging anterolaterally from the brainstem in the cerebellopontine angle. It has vestibular and cochlear divisions innervating hair cells in vestibular organs (semicircular canals and maculae of the utricle and saccule) and the auditory spiral organ of Corti in the cochlear duct, respectively.

Zona incerta. A small sheet of gray matter interposed between the subthalamic nucleus and thalamus, enveloped by efferent fibers of the globus pallidus. The zona incerta has widespread connections, including direct inputs to cerebral cortex, but its function is largely unknown.

Page numbers in **bold** type indicate particularly clear illustrations of a given structure. Page numbers in *italics* indicate a discussion of the structure, either in conjunction with a diagram or in the glossary.